Folk Wisdom
and
Mother Wit

**Recent Titles in
Contributions in Afro-American and African Studies**

A Struggle Worthy of Note: The Engineering and Technological Education of Black Americans
David E. Wharton

African American Soldiers in the National Guard: Recruitment and Deployment During Peacetime and War
Charles Johnson, Jr.

Religion and Suicide in the African-American Community
Kevin E. Early

State Against Development: The Experience of Post-1965 Zaire
Mondonga M. Mokoli

Dusky Maidens: The Odyssey of the Early Black Dramatic Actress
Jo A. Tanner

Language and Literature in the African American Imagination
Carol Aisha Blackshire-Belay, editor

Visible Ellison: A Study of Ralph Ellison's Fiction
Edith Schor

The Early Black Press in America, 1827 to 1860
Frankie Hutton

The Black Laws in the Old Northwest: A Documentary History
Stephen Middleton

The African Aesthetic: Keeper of the Traditions
Kariamu Welsh-Asante, editor

History and Hunger in West Africa: Food Production and Entitlement in Guinea-Bissau and Cape Verde
Laura Bigman

Financing Health Care in Sub-Saharan Africa
Ronald J. Vogel

Folk Wisdom and Mother Wit

John Lee—An African American Herbal Healer

Arvilla Payne-Jackson
and John Lee

Illustrations by Linda Kempton Armstrong

Foreword by James Duke

Contributions in Afro-American and African Studies,
Number 161

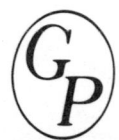

Greenwood Press
Westport, Connecticut • London

Library of Congress Cataloging-in-Publication Data

Payne-Jackson, Arvilla.
   Folk wisdom and mother wit : John Lee—an African American herbal healer / Arvilla Payne-Jackson and John Lee ; illustrations by Linda Kempton Armstrong ; foreword by James Duke.
      p.   cm.—(Contributions in Afro-American and African studies, ISSN 0069-9624 ; no. 161)
   Includes bibliographical references and index.
   ISBN 0-313-28868-2 (alk. paper)
   1. Herbs—North Carolina—Therapeutic use. 2. Lee, John, 1910- . 3. Herbalists—North Carolina. 4. Materia medica, Vegetable—North Carolina. 5. Folk medicine—North Carolina.   I. Lee, John, 1910- . II. Title. III. Series.
RM666.H33P39   1993
615'.321'09756092—dc20
[B]   92-46396

British Library Cataloguing in Publication Data is available.

Copyright © 1993 by Arvilla Payne-Jackson and John Lee

All rights reserved. No portion of this book may be reproduced, by any process or technique, without the express written consent of the publisher.

Library of Congress Catalog Card Number: 92-46396
ISBN: 0-313-28868-2
ISSN: 0069-9624

First published in 1993

Greenwood Press, 88 Post Road West, Westport, CT 06881
An imprint of Greenwood Publishing Group, Inc.

Printed in the United States of America

The paper used in this book complies with the Permanent Paper Standard issued by the National Information Standards Organization (Z39.48-1984).

10 9 8 7 6 5 4 3 2 1

Copyright Acknowledgments

Reprinted with permission from James Duke, *CRC Handbook of Medicinal Plants* (1985), *CRC Handbook of Biologically Active Phytochemicals and Their Activities* (1992), and *CRC Handbook of Phytochemical Constituents of GRAS Herbs and Other Economic Plants* (1992). Copyright CRC Press, Inc., Boca Raton, Fla.

DEDICATED TO

ELIZA JANE SEYMOUR
and
JANE PHILIPS

In the midst of the street of it, and on either side of the river, was there the tree of life which bare twelve manner of fruits, and yielded her fruit every month: and the leaves of the tree were for the healing of the nations.

Revelation 22:2

Contents

Foreword	xi
Acknowledgments	xiii
PART ONE — INTRODUCTION	1
Chapter 1: Historical Overview of African American Folk Medicine	7
Chapter 2: Becoming an Herbalist	17
Chapter 3: Diagnostic System	21
Chapter 4: Classification of the Materia Medica and Illustrations	27
PART TWO — HERBAL REPERTOIRE	35
Appendix: Biologicals	159
References	161
Index	169

Foreword

Arvilla Payne-Jackson came to my office in 1982 requesting assistance in identifying her collection of plants used in folk medicine. The specimens were about the saddest I had ever seen. They were moldy and loosely separated on sheets of note paper torn from a spiral binder. This was a great comfort to me because to this day, colleagues in my peer group make fun of me for my miserable early collections. I am happy to report that both of us have improved and Arvilla has developed near-professional competence. Identification of the herbs was simple enough and the recorded folk usages were consonant with general knowledge of medicinal properties. There was, however, the added dimension of insight into the lives and practices of folk healers and rural usage of home remedies.

My own original work had been directed toward my doctoral dissertation, "Pisammophytes of the Carolina Sandhills" (an abbreviated title), a study of the plants in this interesting environment, which was completed thirty years after the Depression. How sorry I am that I did not meet Mr. John Lee at that time. I would have devoted even more of my efforts to the study of medicinal plants. Finally meeting Mr. Lee at a symposium entitled "The Carolina Connection" at The American University in 1987, I would have introduced him rather than followed him at the podium. I relished the wisdom and humor in his earthy delivery, a hard act to follow. Together on this panel, the African American herbalist and the European American botanist both talked about a subject in which they ardently believed, the curative powers of plants.

There were no real surprises for me in meeting and appreciating Mr. Lee. Dr. Payne-Jackson had introduced me to his thinking over the last few years. I was so interested in her subject that I was happy to pour over her specimens, common names, and field notes, sifting through all the chits to arrive at the right scientific name for the elements in Mr. Lee's pharmacopoeia. I wanted to do all in my power to help record as much as possible about the folk uses of plants, properly identified and vouchered. Now Dr. Payne-Jackson's specimens and the identifications are at least closer to perfect, if not perfect.

With this interesting book, Dr. Payne-Jackson documents yet another folk treasure, the stories of the more important plants used by Mr. Lee in his generous attempts to help cure and treat those who could not afford the silver bullets of modern medicine.

The modern ethnobotanical data in this book are treasures that might have been lost, had not the interrogator and the consultant been both patient, painstaking, and persevering. As a result we have a written record of the folk pharmacopoeia of some lovely sandhill African Americans of the Carolinas, great people from a great part of the world.

There is much more to this book than the folk medicinal applications of plants, but my narrow scientific background will be offered as my excuse for not commenting at length on some of the other interesting folklore recounted herein.

I am glad Mr. Lee kept talking as Dr. Payne-Jackson kept writing, entering into the written record that sort of information that is too often lost, when a healer steps down with no heir apparent.

While there are interesting accounts of native belief about the functioning of the human body, on everything from the poles of the hexes to the roles of the sexes in rural medicine, I comment only on my favorite subject, medicinal plants.

We used to snicker about such concepts as gathering by the moon, collecting from the north side of the tree, avoiding what smelled bad, and so forth, but I can easily see scientific rationales for some of Mr. Lee's beliefs. And I could enumerate dozens of cases where science has found a rationale for the use to which Mr. Lee puts one or another of the plants he uses as medicines. But, I will not.

All human beings all over the earth tend to give their ancestors credit for figuring out which of the plants in their environments were edible and which were poisonous. Why then, today, are we so reluctant to give them credit for being just as wise in selecting the medicinal plants? It seems as if every time I see percentages on the number of folk medicines proving to contain an effective ingredient they lie between 25 percent and 50 percent. I suspect that if the drug companies did one tenth as well in their batting averages, more people could afford their products.

I am pleased to write this brief foreword for this book, a faithful accounting of the honest beliefs of an honest practitioner.

James Duke
Economic Botany
U.S. Department of Agriculture

Acknowledgments

I want to thank all of those who have helped with this book. First and foremost, I thank John Lee and Hattie Mae Lee, who have given so much of their time and shared so much of their lives with me in order to make this book possible, and their children, who have encouraged the recording of their parents' wisdom. I am also deeply grateful to my mentor, colleague, and friend, Dr. Jane Philips, who introduced me to the field of medical anthropology, who made some of the early trips to the Southeast Lowlands with me, and who has given countless hours of guidance and help over the years.

I deeply appreciate and owe a debt of gratitude to Dr. James Duke of the United States Department of Agriculture for freely giving me many hours of help and guidance in the identification of the herbs and for opening his files and resources to me. I am also deeply indebted to Linda Armstrong for the time and talent she has contributed to making the illustrative line drawings included in this book.

My thanks also go to a number of colleagues and friends who have encouraged me in my work over the years and read various versions of this book: Dr. Gertrude Marlowe, Dr. James Scott, Dr. Arnold Taylor, Dr. James Gardiner, and Dr. Ralph Gomes, Mrs. Miriam Pujals, Dr. Elizabeth Espadas, and Mr. Fleming Mathews.

A special thanks to my mother, Virginia Durrant, my aunt and uncle, Anne and Harold Shahan, my sister, Carolyn Bailey, and my friends Margaret and Maurice Thomas, Juan and Elizabeth Espadas, Miriam and Louis Pujals, John and Jeanne Anderegg, and Fleming and Carole Mathews for all of their support. I also give thanks to my husband, Roy, and my children, Meagan and Michael, with deep appreciation for the sacrifices they have made in order to give me the time to complete my work.

Arvilla Payne-Jackson

Acknowledgments

We wish to thank everyone who helped make this book a reality, especially Dr. Arvilla Payne-Jackson, co-author of this book, whose efforts we deeply appreciate. We are most grateful to our niece, Margaret Bryant Pollard, Director of Public Health and Wellness for the Wake Area Health Education Center in Raleigh, North Carolina, and Clinical Assistant Professor, Department of Health Education, University of North Carolina School of Public Health in Chapel Hill, who encouraged us to go public with our knowledge of herbal medicine. She helped us begin our public work with invitations to make presentations at the Wake County Medical Center in Raleigh, North Carolina; the North Carolina Society for the Public Health Education at Camp Caraway, Asheboro, North Carolina; the Folk Health Seminar, at Moncure, North Carolina; the North Carolina Health Convocation at Greensboro, North Carolina; and the Durham County General Hospital, in Durham, North Carolina.

We also want to extend a special thanks to Jack Santino, Glenn Hinson, and Barbara Strickland of the Folklife Museum Program, Museum of History and Technology, Washington, D.C., and to the Smithsonian Institution, who twice invited us to make presentations.

We thank Dr. Brett Williams at The American University, who sponsored the "Carolina-Washington Connection" in Washington, D.C., and invited us to make a presentation. She is the editor of the book *Politics of Culture,* published by the Smithsonian Institution Press, which includes two articles that are earlier presentations of this work: "African American Folk Medicine in the Southeast Lowlands of the United States" (by Dr. Payne-Price) and "John Lee: An African American Healer" (by John Lee and Arvilla Payne-Price).

We also want to extend our thanks for their encouragement to Margaret Marlin from Chewning Junior High School in Durham, North Carolina; George and Lanier Holt with the North Carolina Folklife Festival in Durham, North Carolina; Dr. James Duke of the United States Department of Agriculture; Carolyn Portier, a freelance writer in Chapel Hill, North Carolina; Peggy Payne, a freelance writer in Raleigh, North Carolina; and Brian Shelly, who gave technical assistance.

We also thank the University of North Carolina School of Public Health, Chapel Hill, North Carolina; Fayetteville State University, Fayetteville, North Carolina; Howard University, Washington, D.C.; and the numerous organizations and institutions that have invited us to share our gifts.

John and Hattie Mae Lee

Folk Wisdom
and
Mother Wit

Part One

Introduction

The research for this book is part of an ongoing study of folk medicine and popular health-care practices in the Southeast Lowlands of Virginia, the Carolinas, and Georgia which was begun by two medical anthropologists from Howard University in 1978.[1] It was on this fieldtrip that Professor Payne-Jackson met Mr. Lee, who is the herbalist in his community, Moncure, North Carolina.

The focus of the project addressed the question of why the use of folk medicine persists. Given the fact that modern medicine is widely available it may be surprising that folk medicine is still pervasive. The primary objectives of the initial research were to explore the validity and parameters of the African American folk medical system (1) to find and to identify types of practitioners such as herbalists, "root doctors," and midwives in popular health care; (2) to interview practitioners to learn about their philosophy and motivation, and their individual systems of diagnosis and treatment; and (3) to compile information about folk materia medica and to collect samples of herbs both cultivated and wild.

In general, the preliminary investigation began with informal conversations, and then, a more formal set of questions was asked. Later, structured interviews were administered to friends and professional acquaintances in Washington, D.C. The first persons interviewed gave introductions to additional respondents, and these in turn developed into networks of contacts in Virginia, North Carolina, South Carolina, and Georgia. A total of ninety-one interviews were recorded on 155 hours of tapes.

It was interesting to find that most interviews began with a person's rejection of the idea of the validity of folk cures and a tendency to write them off as "things the old people used." However, when the interviewers brought up the "scientific specifity" and the "active ingredients" in the old-time remedies and added such examples as the alcohol in onions and aspirin from willow bark, the respondents were less hesitant to admit to the validity of the old-time remedies. They were also interested in the large percentage of the early materia medica which continues to be used in current pharmacopoeia and the way that scientists today are returning to study aspects of old remedies which have been overlooked. After this explanation, the respondents usually dropped the pretense of not knowing much about the subject and became actively involved in contributing to the collection of the remedies.

Six categories of information were elicited: (1) How often do people use traditional therapy? (2) Who taught the respondents (both practitioners and users) about the old-home remedies? (3) Why do people rely on old-home remedies? (4) What cures did the respondents know? (5) What are the perceptions about the general diagnostic system of illnesses? and (6) What are the perceptions of supernatural healing?[2]

This research indicated that the African American folk medical system continues to be a vital part of health-care delivery. Watson drew similar conclusions:

> The widespread development and persistence of traditional medicine among Afro-Americans and their corresponding underutilization of modern medical practitioners are largely traceable to the economic poverty of the Black masses and the social history of racial discrimination and oppression that has assured perpetuation of their poverty, ignorance and poor health. (1984:53)

Access to medical facilities and health-care benefits in general has been limited among the African American population. When treatment and facilities were available and affordable the quality was often inadequate and discriminatory. This accounts for the fact that many African Americans, primarily those of the working class and those who live in rural or depressed urban areas, still rely on the old "tried and true" treatments of home remedies. Folk practitioners continue to treat not only physical ailments but also mental, interpersonal, and spiritual disorders (cf. Watson 1984:1; Mathews et al. 1992:8-9).

Many African Americans still use folk medicine because it meets both physiological and psychological needs as interpreted within their socio-cultural setting. Blaustein (1992:36) points out, "traditional healers often display effective practical knowledge of psychological and emotional needs of their patients which leads to successful healing on various levels." (See also Bannerman et al. 1983; McQuire 1988.)

Raboteau suggests some reasons that folk medicine became and continues to be pervasive in the African American community:

> Given the poverty of many black Americans and the high cost of medical care, given the cultural distance between black communities and predominantly white medical facilities, given the lack of rapport between black patients and white medical professionals, it is not

surprising that alternate forms of healing became important for African Americans. (1986:555)

The extent of choice is limited for the financially disadvantaged people in both towns and rural areas. They take advantage of the availability of a relatively inexpensive health-care system which offers various types of folk medicine, such as herbs and patent medicines, which are nonprescription medicines that can be purchased from herbal shops and drug stores. Folk medicine also provides a personal element that scientific medicine may overlook. While folk medicine is valued predominantly by the old, the poor, and working-class African Americans, a new clientele is developing which includes young and middle-class people living in both rural and urban areas. This is the result, in part, of the perceived inadequacy and mistrust of scientific medicine (de Albuquerque 1979:38).

The question proposed at the outset of this research was, Why does folk medicine persist today? The pervasive preference for the old traditions as opposed to scientifically advanced biomedical care involves factors which go far beyond the economic motive. The people are more comfortable with traditions which are compatible with their own cultural perceptions and experiences than they are with the unfamiliar and often considered depersonalized application of modern medicine. This is particularly true in clinical practice. The personal element is more evident in the interpersonal network of recommendations and referrals in folk medicine than in the mainstream process of referral of patients to doctors. The more personalized referral in folk medicine develops a significant degree of trust.

An additional source of outside-of-the-family resources in times of trouble and illness is the loosely structured system of neighborhood "natural helping networks" (Collins and Pancoast 1976?). Such networks arise as extensions of the primary healing resources for coping or as alternatives to the customary reliance on families. In fact, the social alternatives increase the therapeutic choices. Watson (1984:64), commenting on Durkheim's (1956) analysis of social historical change in ways of life, points out that "there will be limits set by tradition on the extent to which novel forms of medical technology will be introduced and accepted in a society."

Two increasingly frequent terms in the anthropological studies of change in medical habits are "medical pluralism" and "alternative medicine." Hughes suggests that the decline of disease and the successes of biomedicine lead the public to change to the modern system (1968:160). Watson (1984:64), however, points out that "the respect shown by older . . . patients for modern medical practices is conditioned by the beliefs about health care current in the society where the patients live."

In "Concepts and a Model for the Comparison of Medical Systems as Cultural Systems," Kleinman suggests that there are three areas of medicine:

popular, professional, and folk; this division necessitates decisions and choice (1978:86). For example, the perceived cause of illness is a factor in choice of treatment. Availability, both logistic and monetary, is another factor. Both the syncretic therapy and the integrated ethnic healing systems are classified as "pluralistic." This "pluralism" increases the area of choice.

Watson adds: "Choice of herbal medicine may be associated with an absence of modern medical facilities in the local area, a lack of knowledge about alternative kinds of health care, segregation of newer or local facilities, and real or expected discrimination in patient referrals to modern medical doctors" (1984:57).

The similarity of responses obtained in the interviews conducted in the five states during the fieldwork validated the presumed existence of an African American health-care system. The utilization of this system is directly correlated to age, social class, education, and residence location (urban/rural). While older, poorer, and less educated African Americans are likely to rely on the folk medical system, both knowledge and use of it extend to some degree into all of the other classes.

As stated at the outset, the plan was to identify types of practitioners. At the beginning of this study, a practical nurse from the Moncure Community Health Clinic introduced us to Mr. and Mrs. Lee. We spent the better part of the day with the family; we also toured the Lee cultivated herb garden and walked through the surrounding natural woods and fields. We collected samples of plants and herbs used in Mr. Lee's extensive ethnobotanical practice. Both Mr. Lee and Mrs. Lee serve not only the local community but also clients from coast to coast. Mr. Lee is the primary practitioner and Mrs. Lee specializes in the area of childhood and female complaints. Mr. Lee collects most of the herbs and Mrs. Lee helps with their preparation. When clients are unable to visit they write to Mr. Lee for advice. The Lees have contributed their experience and knowledge to various local, state, and national panels on health care; two folk medical programs at the Smithsonian Institution in 1979 and 1991; and presentations at various hospitals and universities.

Mr. Lee was the most highly trained and experienced practitioner interviewed during the initial fieldwork. He was generous with his time and information. He is part of the traditional African American folk medical system. He uses elements of biomedicine, adapting them to the frame of reference of the older traditions. His willingness to share his knowledge comes from a deep conviction of the importance of the continuation of the folk wisdom and mother wit passed down from previous generations.

The fundamental role played by the Lees in the practical health care system may be better understood in the general context of the African American folk medical system. Chapter 1 gives a brief overview of the historical setting of African American folk medicine. The second chapter describes how the Lees became involved in the healing arts. Chapter 3 describes the diagnostic system used by Mr. Lee in his practice. Chapter 4 provides a discussion of the materia medica and some illustrations. Some of the immediate herbal information is summarized in Part Two. This last section gives sixty of the ethnobotanicals most commonly used by Mr. Lee. The Appendix provides a list of some non-botanical materials used in folk medicine.

NOTES

1. This work was made possible partly by support from the faculty research program in the Social Sciences, Humanities and Education at Howard University from the Office of the Vice President of Academic Affairs, 1979-80. This initial research was undertaken with Dr. Jane Philips, my colleague at Howard University. On subsequent field trips, students were offered the opportunity of fieldwork training for credit.

2. For a discussion of the results of the fieldwork see A. Payne-Price, "African American Folk Medicine in the Southeast Lowlands of the United States," in Brett Williams, ed., *The Politics of Culture,* Washington, D.C.: Smithsonian Institution Press, 1991, 133-153.

Chapter 1

Historical Overview of African American Folk Medicine

This book is intended to serve as a general introduction to the African American folk-medical system. One facet of this is illustrated in a description of the herbal practice of John Lee. Mr. Lee is a completely dedicated herbal practitioner who has many times expressed his ideal of service to the community. He has declared that if he felt that he were not helping people, he would abandon his practice. This first chapter provides a brief historical setting for Mr. Lee's philosophy and practice. His work is within the African American folk-medical system, which has identifiable characteristics built on a core of perceptions and practices. This central core developed from an amalgamation of intercultural theoretical and practical approaches (European colonial, African, American Indian) and a combination of the differing medicines. Snow defines this system as:

> a composite of classical medicine of an earlier day, European folklore regarding the natural world, rare African traits,[1] and selected beliefs derived from modern scientific medicine. The whole is inextricably blended with the tenets of fundamentalist Christianity, elements of the Voodoo religion of the West Indies, and the added spice of sympathetic magic. It is a coherent system and not a ragtag collection of isolated superstition. (1974:83)[2]

The evolution of African American folk medicine began with the cultural contact and borrowing among European colonial, African slave, and American Indian cultures. This merging brought into practice the adaptation and combined application of the various medical systems and practices in the southeastern coastlands and colonies (Kiev 1968; Mitchell 1978; Watson 1984).

Early European settlers enlarged the general health practices by this combination. The Old World components included notions of etiology and perceptions of therapy. Etiologies included Kirchner's animalculaer particles; Claudius Galen's theory on humoral imbalances of the four humors (blood, phlegm, yellow bile and black bile); and Thomas Sydenham's theory that morbific substances "released by decay, infected the air and entered the body through the respiratory tract" (Otto 1984:69). The therapeutic practices were largely based on purging, vomiting, bloodletting, trephanning, blistering, and sweating. The settlers brought their native herbs and simples and added American Indian and African American botanicals to their own (Vogel 1970; Hamel and Chiltoskey 1975; Mitchell 1978; Croom 1992). While medical botanicals are the most widely recognized contribution American Indians made to the colonial pharmacopoeia, they also contributed their practices of sweat baths and massage. The African contributions in the "Low Country" which includes North Carolina are described by Berlin (1980:56):

> The transplanted African's intimate knowledge of the subtropical lowland environment—especially when compared to the Englishman's dense ignorance—magnified white dependence on blacks. . . . Since the geography, climate, and topography of the low-country more closely resembled the West African than the English countryside, African not European technology and agronomy often guided lowland development. From the first, whites depended on blacks to identify useful flora and fauna and to define the appropriate methods of production. . . . In short, transplanted Englishmen learned as much or more from transplanted Africans as did the former African from them . . . both whites and blacks incorporated much of West African culture into their new way of life.

Postell (1951) reviewed various plantation owners' records, diaries, and correspondence in an effort to understand the health status of plantation slaves. Some of the general illnesses they suffered during slavery were "cholera, pneumonia, dysentery, certain dietary deficiency diseases and probably to a lesser extent than his white master, from yellow fever and malaria."[3] Swados (1941) examined historical documents and determined that plantation slaves suffered from a number of illnesses which did not appear to afflict the white plantation owners. Duffy (1968) attributed the living conditions of the slaves as the primary source of the types of illnesses common to slaves.

Deas-Moore (1987:476) provides a socio-environmental summary of the slaves' health: "the Africans' new environment presented new health problems. The incidence of respiratory diseases, tuberculosis, hypertension, lactose intolerance and many infectious diseases . . . was probably facilitated by new dietary habits and cramped living conditions."

Plantation owners and their overseers, safeguarding the economic investment in the work force, provided the primary medical care on the plantations. Local physicians, books, and journals served as sources of advice about disease causation and therapy (Otto 1984:114-15). Physicians, retained by owners, were used to attend the slaves, primarily during times of epidemics or acute illnesses.

Historical Overview

Medical practitioners in the eighteenth and nineteenth centuries, besides the copious use of drugs, resorted almost entirely to bleeding and blistering, measures which weakened the patient or aggravated his suffering. Emetics, purgatives, opiates and barks formed the materia medica and could be dispensed by anyone, along with home remedies from herbs and tonics, whiskey and brandy. (Anderson 1985:106)

Rosengarten describes the medical relations on plantations in South Carolina as "relations of force."

> The threat of calling the doctor was enough to drive some hands out of the sickhouse and into the fields, because they feared the doctor would find nothing wrong with them or because they feared his treatment. Blacks tried first to cure themselves, with teas, powders, and salves made from local plants and animals; with charms, prayer and conjuration-magic. Drugs alone, they believed, could not restore good health. Only by conciliating an evil spirit loosed by an enemy, living or dead, could a person overcome illness. If herbal remedies and magic failed, the patient's condition might be desperate by the time the master was notified. Once seen by the doctor, the patient had to be closely watched if he or she was to follow the doctor's instructions. Planters wanted to think of their slaves as unwilling children who had to be made to take their castor oil. The slaves wanted to control their own bodies and souls. Their attitude suggests the existence of an alternative theory of disease. But whites in general showed no interest in the blacks' ideas of causation, which Chaplin typically dismissed as "foolishness." (1986:187)

Because of the lack of physicians and inadequate care by the owners, the slaves assumed a major role in nursing the ill slaves, the masters, and their families. Mitchell (1978:13;15) points out that from an early period, "Afro-Americans were involved in health-related activities. . . . Slaves maintained their own medical practices especially to cure everyday illnesses" because of the neglect of owners and overseers.

Savitt (1978:173-74) also describes the medical practices of slaves in antebellum times. Selected slaves dispensed "white" remedies, and participated in obstetrics, as well as bloodletting, extracting teeth, administering medicine, and caring for the sick.

In addition to the conventional approach, the slave had become well versed in the herbal and root medicines on the plantation. Some slaves recognized the botanical relationship of the plantation genera to the African genera, for example, pennyroyal and belladonna. They had their own practitioners, the best known being the conjure doctors. In fact, conjuring was the basis of the supernaturally induced illnesses and troubles. This covered a wide spectrum ranging from the gripes to infidelity. The plantation owners themselves rejected the slaves' ideas of supernatural causes of disease and condemned and forbade the practice of the hoodoo, voodoo, and witchcraft. Records, nevertheless, indicate that they themselves secretly resorted to the conjure doctors (Hyatt 1970-78).

Throughout slavery and up to the present day, there were culturally patterned sets of ideas about causes of illnesses and injuries. The causes and cures that existed are divided into two basic categories: natural and unnatural (Foster 1976; Mitchell 1978; Watson 1984; Deas-Moore 1987). Natural illness explains "illness in impersonal systemic terms. Disease is thought to stem ... from such *natural forces or conditions* as cold, heat, winds, dampness, and above all, by an upset in the balance of the basic body elements" (Foster 1976:775). Unnatural illness falls into two subcategories (Mitchell 1978; Watson 1984): (1) *occult illness,* which is caused by evil spirits; by the use of sorcery by "root doctors" or "conjurers," and (2) *spiritual illness,* which is the penalty incurred for sins or "caused by God." Occult and spiritual illnesses can affect both the physical and the spiritual health of an individual.

These perceptions of causes of illness and injury stem from the age-old concepts found in the ancestral homelands of the slaves. Raboteau (1986) discusses the role of religion, including worldview, magic, and medicine, in the interaction of the health and disease of the slaves. He underscores this interaction in the socio-cultural dynamics of family and community within the natural surroundings. Illness was associated with disharmony in the socio-cultural and/or the natural environment. Such illness could be treated with natural herbal remedies, but religious rituals and magical charms were also necessary.

Religion and magic continued to play a central role in the folk-medical health care during slavery. Christian charisma ("shouting churches") with ecstatic spirit possession provided an acceptable alternative for the tradition of spirit possession in African religions. "Catching the spirit" gave status and prestige to the worshiper and his/her community (Raboteau 1986:541-45).

The religious aspect of African American health care included magical ingredients and religious curing ceremonies and rituals. These became known as "conjuring" or the African American "magical medicine." As stated, conjuring accounted for illnesses within the socio-cultural context. The power of conjurers extended over both cause and cure. Raboteau (1986:550) also points out that,

> for a largely powerless people, conjuring functioned as a symbolic assertion of power. Story after story of black folklore celebrated the ability of conjurers to manipulate whites as well as blacks. . . . The contention that the white doctor's medicine was useless against the charms of the black conjurers represented a subtle but effective

rejection of white supremacy in matters medical and magical. And the sight of white clients patiently waiting upon the skills of black conjurers proved the same point (cf. Hyatt 1970-78).

On plantations there was a hierarchy of therapists and treatments: family, herbalists, conjurers, and, if needed, plantation owner and/or physician. The herbalists were knowledgeable about medicinal botanicals and their uses. Some combined these basic medical ingredients with rudimentary but more extensive resources in elementary pharmacopoeia. When these proved ineffective or an illness lingered, a conjurer offered an alternative treatment. The plantation owner or physician was called if the family, herbalist, and conjurer were unsuccessful.

Another type of African American health practitioner was the midwife or "granny midwife." From the days of slavery to recent times they commanded great respect in the community. Midwives not only helped deliver babies but were also responsible for other medical practices on the plantation (Moton 1899). The day-to-day health care of slaves was entrusted to these African American women, who effectively combined their bitter herb and root teas with the medicines left by the physician or dispensed by the mistress (Deas-Moore 1978:482).

Pre-Civil War notions and ideas about illness have continued through economic readjustments that followed the war and are very much in evidence today. The post-Civil War rural economy was based on agriculture with tobacco, cotton, and rice as the primary cash crops. These complexes "utilized the common forms of Southern tenure—owner, tenants and sharecroppers. . . . The elements of paternalism that developed during slavery persisted and increasingly crossed the color line" (Daniel 1985:xii). During this time racially divisive attitudes such as Jim Crow laws and other racially motivated legislation influenced all areas of life, including the quality of medical facilities and health care available to the African Americans.

Within the African American communities there were all too few African American physicians and professionals in the health-care services. However, there was some compensation within the African American community for the poorer quality of health care. The primary sources of help were church activities and organizations, such as sodalities. In addition to the expected help from family members, friends and church members came to the aid of patients during the time of illness. Fraternal orders, such as The Independent Order of Saint Luke, headed by Maggie Walker in Richmond, Virginia, in the first part of the century, offered sickness and death benefits to African Americans.[4] Other continuing practitioners serving the community from plantation days were herbalists, midwives, and conjurers. Itinerant religious healers and the men and women with medicine wagons who sold a variety of herbal and patent medicines formed another branch of alternative services.

These separate forms of health services were necessary because of the existing socio-economic structure and its concomitant racial dichotomy. The racial differentiation established a striking contrast in the available health services. The African American distrust of the European American was justified, and extended into the medical arena as a result of physicians regarding African Americans as inferior and, thereby, justifying the use of slaves for experimentation with new surgical techiniques and treatments. The resulting mistrust is reflected in a statement made in 1979 by Abraham Jenkins, a descendant of the Sea Islands slaves: "How could I develop an attitude of respect for someone who is supposed to be a professional and who has no respect for me?" (Jenkins 1979:11).

Changes in agriculture followed the Depression, industrialization and mechanization of agriculture in the 1950s and 1960s with a decrease in demand for tobacco, cotton, and rice. Consequently, after World War II, there were large migrations of African Americans to urban areas. Clinics and hospitals were more available and offered more comprehensive care than existed in the rural areas; however, the mistrust of the health-care personnel continued. Costs were excessive and this discouraged a more general usage of the modern health-care system.

As education and economic status have risen among African Americans in the latter part of this century, so has their use of modern medicine. Today, it is mostly poor African Americans who use folk medicine as the dependable alternate health resource (Mitchell 1978; Snow 1981; Watson 1984).

In both urban and rural communities the service provided by a network of African American healers continues. This is an extension of the earlier system of networks of folk-medical practitioners. Today, as in earlier times, and in all ethnic groups, the immediate family and elders are the first resource to meet medical needs. When the family or elders are inadequate, practitioners such as herbalists or religious healers may be called upon. The choice will depend partially on the perceived cause of the illness.

An herbalist may be seen as the most appropriate healer for "natural" illnesses. These herbal specialists are usually part-time practitioners, well versed in botanical ways of dealing with health difficulties and problems. Not only do they diagnose and treat illnesses and "ailments," they prepare their own medications. The treatments may be accompanied by rituals. When necessary they assume the role of "folk psychiatrist." Herbalists may be paid in cash or gifts. Some practitioners refuse payment or gifts because of religious convictions which forbid them from accepting any rewards or returns. There is also the belief that accepting payment may result in the loss of their healing powers.

Until recently, lay midwives treated childhood ailments and injuries. In addition to practicing midwifery, they cultivated their own herbs and collected and prepared natural herbal materia medica. Licensing of midwives in the South began during the 1940s primarily for the purpose of teaching hygiene (cf.

Historical Overview

Deas-Moore 1987). They usually apprenticed themselves to doctors or other midwives until they were proficient. They were sometimes paid with money. More frequently they were paid "in kind" with produce or animals. Today lay-midwives have been replaced by nurse-midwives.[5]

If a patient or family feels an illness is "unnatural," either a "root doctor" or a faith healer may be called upon. "Root doctors" or "conjurers" are practitioners who usually require a high fee. They are alleged to be able to use their powers to harm, kill, or cure a person. For the most part, they use charms and potions and magical rituals to put a "fix" or "roots" on people, animals, and things. This latter applies to damaging possessions or processes.[6]

Faith healers, in either church denominations or "store fronts," are the practitoners who call on supernatural forces and by using prayer and "laying-on-of-hands" effect cures for illnesses thought to be of a "spiritual" nature.

Spiritual illness is thought to be caused by either God or Satan. Faith healers treat everyday problems, depression, worry, and general complaints. Donations for their work are expected or required (cf. Mitchell 1978; Primack 1984).

Hall and Bourne (1973) tell of the work of "neighborhood prophets" in Atlanta. These primarily diagnose and treat primarily psycho-social problems through the use of prayers, divine intervention, dreams, and reports of déjà vu by the patients.

There are also three types of supernatural religious healers who have highly specialized roles: those who "talk-out-fire," "talk-out-bleeding," and "talk-off-warts." "Blood-stoppers" have a verbal ritual in which they use individual invocation of supernatural powers by continually repeating Ezekiel 16:6. Warts can be removed by prayer. The prayer is accompanied by making the sign of a cross over the wart using a piece of animal bone to effect supernatural removal. Healers who "talk-out-fire" or burns pray and conduct a ritual act such as blowing over the burned area.

In addition, aspects of modern medicine incorporate the use of over-the-counter medicines. Watson (1984) points out the importance of neighborhood druggists in the folk-medical system.

> Elderly Afro-Americans use a variety of herbs and over-the-counter preparations that appear to be unique to their ethnic group (54). . . . [They also] showed a marked preference for and belief in the efficacy of remedies recommended by local druggists with little or no reference made to the comparative utility of modern medical doctors. (56-57)

Another folk-medical resource found in urban areas is the "magic vendor." Hall and Bourne (1973) describe magic vendors in Atlanta, who sell magic and operate from, or in association with, herbal shops. They specialize in providing health aids, promoting domestic harmony, improving sex life, and providing clients with the means to make more money and to change their destinies.

Nearly all use patent medicines, drugs, health and beauty aids, and magical religious objects, symbols, or substances to achieve their ends.

The African American folk-medical system and healers like Mr. Lee are an integral part of the health care system in both rural and urban communities.

Economically marginal rural and urban African Americans in need of medical services may utilize the more accessible alternative health-care system because it is less costly than modern biomedicine, more personal, and more compatible with their perceptions of disease etiology and treatment.

Mathews (1992:7-8) describes the bleak picture of the health-care system that exists in North Carolina. She attributes the rise of self-reliance for health care and the use of alternative medical systems to a combination of socio-ecological conditions in North Carolina: geographic isolation in rural areas, lack of educational opportunities, limited or no access to government services, and extreme poverty. The lack of biomedical health-care personnel only exacerbates the situation. Wilms and Powell (1983:17, as cited in Mathews et al. 1992) reported that the ratio of doctors to patients in thirty-two eastern North Carolina counties varied from 1:539 in urban areas to 1:3550 in predominantly African American inland counties to none at all in at least three counties.

Mathews et al. (1992) reports the results of a survey conducted with 900 older adults randomly sampled by race, ethnic group, and gender across twelve counties in eastern North Carolina. The preliminary results indicate that in general 35 percent of the population surveyed use "some form of traditional or alternative medicine, most often in conjunction with some form of biomedicine" (8).[7] The highest percentage of use, between 50 and 60 percent, was found in the African American community. The use of folk medicine by many of the African American people in North Carolina only points out the importance of incorporation of the folk realm into the biomedical realm of medicine to serve the needs of patients better and to prevent cultural conflicts which are likely to arise between the two systems of diagnosis and treatment (Saunders 1953; Haufman 1979).

NOTES

1. The Voodoo religion is actually part of the West African systems of ancestor veneration and animism.

2. In Snow's definition of the African American folk-medical system she refers to the "African traits" as rare. Our research, however, shows that the African contribution is more extensive. Not only did the Africans contribute to their own health care, but many of their points of view and beliefs were incorporated into the larger colonial system. They also added to the knowledge of the ethnobotany and medicine and in some cases contributed actual specimens (cf. Grime 1976; Ayensu 1978).

Historical Overview

3. The relationship between sickle cell trait and immunity to malaria has recently been discovered and partly explains the lower incidence of malaria among the slaves.

4. Marlowe (1987).

5. Nurse-midwives today are being driven out of business by high malpractice insurance costs.

6. One informant gave this explanation for the difference between root doctors and conjurers: A conjure man and a root doctor are almost the same thing. "It works kind a together. . . . The way I see it, a conjurer, they mostly jus' put it down for you, and you be sick if you step over it. . . . A root doctor, he jus' fix up medicine for you . . . maybe in bottles, or put it in little sacks for you and things like potions or charms, an' name it, causin' you to hurt."

7. An important point made by Murphee (1970) is that patients who use folk remedies do not report the use to their doctors. One point of concern here is that the herbal tea or home remedy may actually contain active ingredients which may interfere with screening or testing for particular diseases.

Chapter 2

Becoming an Herbalist

Mr. Lee as an herbalist and healer is a nationally recognized practitioner. His practice is representative of Southern herbalists'. He has come into his practice by learning from the members of his family, who were already established as healers for over a hundred years.

Members of the community consider Mr. Lee, his family, and their services an important part of their health care. He is knowledgeable about the local herbs and their practical effectiveness. Mr. Lee's knowledge of botany extends beyond his experience with local plants. He refers to such classic sources as Jethro Kloss's *Back to Eden*, *The Herbalist* by Joseph Meyer, *Growing and Using the Healing Herbs* by Gaea Weiss and Shandar Weiss, *The Herb Book* by John Lust, and *Magic and Medicine of Plants* published by Reader's Digest Association. He is familiar with the work of James Duke, who works for the United States Department of Agriculture and participated with him on a panel on "The North Carolina Connection" at American University in 1987. He himself has contributed to the literature in the field.[1]

His training began with helping his mother, Eliza Jane Seymour, when he was a child. She was a midwife. Her knowledge drew on traditions of her mixed American Indian (Lumbo/Cherokee), Irish/British, and African descent.

She learned her basic healing arts from her own mother, who was of Indian descent. She served all ethnic groups in Chatham and Lee counties. She not only delivered children but also treated childhood as well as adult illnesses.

Mr. Lee would accompany his mother when she was helping women with childbirth or families who had an ill member. If she had the need of some particular herb, she would send him to get it.

Out of these experiences he developed a sense of the community health-care system. When a person became ill the first resort was the family. If the illness extended over a long period, other family units would freely volunteer their services and assistance for anywhere from one day to a few weeks. These services included helping with work on the farm and household chores such as laundry, cooking, and cleaning. If the medical needs seemed to extend beyond the familiar old-home remedies, the skills of the midwives, herbalists, and "root doctors" were invoked. The physician was the last resort and was called only when a person seemed to be "going backwards." This was considered necessary when a high fever lingered or constantly recurred.

Out of his work with his mother Mr. Lee learned not only basic health care and medical practices but also the rudiments of the local medical botany. He learned which botanicals to use for different illnesses, where to collect them, and how to prepare them. His father, Thomas Lee, contributed to his herbal training as well and was also famous for his supernatural ability to "talk-out-fire" and "talk-out-bleeding."

Mr. Lee, himself, was considered to have a special gift. He was born with a caul or "veil" over his face, which is believed to convey special perceptions and abilities. Healers who have been born with a veil are thought to have insights, and special diagnostic abilities and remedies for difficult health problems.

Mr. Lee's mother died in 1928. The community people still sought out the family for help and treatment because the nearest doctor was over twelve miles away. At that time transportation was either by foot or by mule. Maude, Mr. Lee's sister, continued her mother's midwifery practice. John and his older brother, Tom, developed their own herbal practice. There was often a continuum of family medical data. Tom added new health practices which he learned while working in the coal mines of West Virginia.

When Mr. Lee married, he found employment out of the community. He would return home on weekends and continued to help the neighbors and local people. He retired in the early 1970s, at which time his practice was not only fully renewed but expanded. It was then that his wife, Hattie Mae, joined him as a full partner in his practice.

In the early years Hattie Mae Lee did not participate in the practice because basically she did not believe in the efficacy of the herbal remedies. She would, however, make some teas for her children. For example, she would use catnip (*Nepeta cataria*) tea to help settle their stomachs. It was not until Mr. Lee cured her of a bad case of poison ivy by using the crushed leaves and berries of nightshade (*Solanum nigrum*) that Hattie Mae changed her mind. She told how it happened.

> I went down to the river to fish. I stood there awhile until I started to get tired. Someone had chopped out a place, so I sat down, not thinking about bothering me. When I got back home, the back of my legs and the bends of my knees were all red. I had broken out in poison ivy. At that time my husband was working away from home at the saw mill. When he came home, I was walking kind of stiff-legged. He said, "What is wrong with you?" I said, "I went fishing and got poison ivy." He got some nightshade and told me to bruise the leaves

and berries and put them in a piece of cloth and then put it in milk and bathe the back of my legs. In a day or two I could hardly tell I had it. So then I began to pay a little more attention.

This was the beginning of Hattie Mae's taking a serious role in her husband's work. She has taken on the primary responsibility of preparing the herbal remedies. Another role she has is to conduct the interviews with women who complain of "female problems." She then consults Mr. Lee about the appropriate treatment.

In summary, the Lees feel that their knowledge of the herbs is a gift from God to be used to help and to serve people. Mr. Lee puts it succinctly: "After I see I have helped people, I feel justified in getting these herbs for them, because I have the feeling of helping them. It's good to have knowledge and if you don't use what you have, you might as well bury it. The Lord helps me with this treating."

Both the Lees believe that God gave a specific plant to cure each illness.

> The Lord put these things here and that's what we use. Scripture says bitter herbs have more medicinal value. In the beginning that was all we had to use. We didn't have the pills and all the things we have now and even the people who used to sell patent medicines used to fix it in the bottles and carry it around and sell it.

The Lees see that there are various types of illnesses. There are two main divisions. The first is physical and caused by "nature." These illnesses include infections, such as colds, measles, and bronchitis, caused by microorganisms, and the trauma of accidents. The second is psychological, including such phenomena as "nervous breakdown," severe depression, and "mental disturbances." In this latter category "supernatural" afflictions and "possession" are excluded. The Lees only treat illnesses that are classified as natural.

Originally, the Lees worked with their own family members. Therapeutic services were also rendered to some friends outside the family and eventually spread to the larger community. Today, referrals came from all points of the United States. Specific information about the way Mr. Lee diagnoses illnesses follows in the next chapter.

NOTE

1. John Lee and Arvilla Payne-Price, "John Lee: An African American Herbal Healer," in Brett Williams, ed., *The Politics of Culture* (Washington, D.C.: Smithsonian Institution Press, 1991), pp. 155-71.

Chapter 3

Diagnostic System

The diagnostic system of African American folk medicine places primary importance on blood and the balance of binary qualities associated with generation, volume, location, circulation, viscosity, purity, and temperature. Phlegm is a secondary diagnostic component in the determination of health. Intercultural exchanges explain regional differences in the diagnostic systems. According to Snow (1977:34) who made a study of African American folk medicine in Arizona:

> Of the original humors, blood and phlegm are the components which receive the most attention. Heat is still associated with blood which thickens to keep one warm in the winter, with fevers, and skin eruptions. Cold is associated with phlegm . . . with damp air and water. . . . The greatest attention, however, is focused on blood. It is probably the most important single factor to be considered in the maintenance of good health. The state of the blood is an index of the state of the system, and may vary along several dimensions. If any general statement can be made about the blood it is that it is never static—responding to a variety of external and internal stimuli, the blood goes "up" and "down," is "high" or "low," "clean" or "defiled," "good" or "bad."

In Mr. Lee's system the following binary qualities are used to describe the state of the blood: good/bad (blood purity), fast/slow (circulation), high/low (quantity/location), hot/cold (temperature), and thick/thin (viscosity). When a person is ill there is an imbalance in one or more of these factors. Mr. Lee assesses various symptoms to determine which imbalance of qualities may be causing the illness.

BLOOD PURITY: GOOD/BAD

People with "good blood" do not suffer much illness. They do not have many colds. Diabetes, venereal disease, and blood poisoning are the three major causes of "bad blood." These are thought to be impurities that must be cleansed from the body. Sores that do not heal quickly and passing blood are two indications of "bad blood."

Mr. Lee uses these symptoms and, in addition, on examination, asks if the patient has experienced such other problems as "falling out" (fainting), dizzy spells, fits, and spasms. The condition of the skin is another significant indicator. A general irritation such as "scaly," "dead," or "fuzzy looking" skin may signify bad blood.

BLOOD QUANTITY/LOCATION: HIGH/LOW

A patient who is said to have "high blood" is considered to have either too much blood or most of the blood located in the upper part of the body. The blood is believed to go up to the head, where it "slows down and collects [and] does not work its way down again."[1] A person with high blood pressure has "too much blood." A change in diet is advised. Modification includes cutting down on or eliminating entirely certain foods, such as pork, seafood, fried chicken or meat with fat on it, starchy foods, coffee, and whiskey. Other foods are recommended to build up the blood, for example, liver. A person with "low blood" has insufficient blood and it is not circulating or "going up" into the body as it should.

Three indicators used to determine whether blood is high or low are: (1) impaired vision and "bleariness" of the eyes, (2) pain in the head and eyes, sometimes accompanied by "falling out," and (3) the appearance of the veins in the crook of the arm and back of the hand.

A person with high or low blood has "blurry feelings" about the head, his eyes and head "hurt a lot," or she is susceptible to "visions or flashes on and off." Swollen and/or raised veins in the crook of the arm and the back of the hand indicate high blood. High blood also causes greater susceptiblity to fever. Sluggishness, lethargy, and lack of energy characterize a person with low blood. If blood is low in quantity, a proper diet including beef and iron is prescribed. An imbalance of the blood in terms of location is treated by infusions and extracts to make the blood "hot." This speeds up the circulation, which reestablishes the balance sooner.

BLOOD CIRCULATION: FAST/SLOW

In contrast to the classical humoral theory, in which seasonal change was associated with types of disease, the African American folk-medical system associates changes in weather with the circulation of blood, which in turn affects health. The speed of the blood flow "acts like a pair of scales and needs to be kept in balance."

Mr. Lee thinks blood circulation changes with the seasons. Blood is thought to move from slow/cool in the winter to fast/warm in the summer. According to Mr. Lee "a person is like a tree: the sap is in the roots and only starting to rise in the spring, so a person is weaker. By winter a person is built up."

Temperature can affect the blood circulation and can influence susceptibility to illness. Continued low temperature of the blood can cause it to be "slow." A person with slow blood circulation is vulnerable to colds, arthritis, fits, and spasms. A person with slow blood "just feels slouchy." When the blood slows down, so does the individual. When a vein does not open normally, it can cause blood to "pile up," resulting in a blood clot or stroke. The blood reaches a certain spot and reverses its flow.

Slow blood is low; high blood is fast. Activity speeds up the heart, causing a faster circulation and higher blood temperature. High fast blood is considered to be hot because "it is going to the brain and not coming back."

BLOOD TEMPERATURE: HOT/COLD

In summary, the speed of the blood flow is affected by the interaction of the functions associated with fast/hot and slow/cold. Fast movement increases the blood temperature; slow movement cools the blood temperature. A healthy person needs to maintain a proper balance. Mr. Lee determines the blood temperature by asking the patient about his or her reactions to the feelings of hot and cold and their duration.

Continuing comfortable warmth indicates health. Hot blood causes rashes, and cold blood is associated with respiratory ailments, colds, and arthritis.

BLOOD VISCOSITY: THICK/THIN

Blood viscosity corresponds to blood temperature and circulation. Thick blood flows slowly, building up the degree of pressure. The improper circulation clogs up the veins. A stroke or brain damage may result. An active medicine such as epsom salts thins the blood. Mr. Lee says that the thickness of blood is difficult to determine unless a person has a cut or sore. Lee goes on to say, "Thick blood makes blood high because it is not flowing—it is slow moving because it's cold."

Mr. Lee recognizes the two types of blood cells, red and white. Thin blood indicates an imbalance between the two. "One is taking more [calories] than the other and it is not moving through the body as it should." Low thin blood or "tired blood" may be corrected through change in diet.

The categories of thick/thin and hot/cold are interdependent. Age and sex correlate with these sets. Babies have thin blood; this thickens in maturity but begins to become thin again around the age of fifty-five or sixty. This low thin blood of elderly people accounts for their feeling the cold more keenly.

Women are believed to have a greater supply of thicker blood than men. Consequently, they can withstand cold temperature better. An increase in blood flow may be caused by getting wet and chilled during menses as a result of bathing, washing hair, or overrapid cooling. And Mr. Lee says that women are able to regenerate blood lost through menses. Men cannot regenerate lost blood.

Today there is a proliferation of media information on the specialization of the bilateral functions of the human brain. Mr. Lee condenses these concepts. "Half of the brain is for thinking and all the things that come in the mind, and the other half is for the nerves." Each half plays a specific role. If there is an imbalance in the system many things can happen to a person. For example, "Most people have a stroke on the left side which is the thinking part—the blood piles up and causes an imbalance."

PHLEGM

Mr. Lee believes that phlegm is the second most important factor in determining health. He says that "phlegm is already in a person" and when a person is exposed to and inhales damp cold air the temperature permeates the body.

"The phlegm ['darkness'] and cold air get into the intestines or around them or in the side or back." If the blood is cold and slow it hinders the circulation. This phlegm then gets into the lungs and causes congestion and wheezing. From the extended exposure to cold and wet, phlegm may cause a reaction in the system. It continues to collect until the person catches a cold. Mr. Lee listens to the cough and observes how the person spits. This determines the degree of congestion in the lungs and chest.

GALL

The gall and liver help regulate the body by eliminating impurities. According to Mr. Lee, the "gall," attached to the liver, produces bile, which aids in digestion of food. A person with gall or liver problems complains of a "foul" or "sour" stomach. Food tastes bitter and "the mouth is not clear in either talking or breath."

OTHER DIAGNOSTIC ELEMENTS

Mr. Lee uses numerous other diagnostic elements in his system. He has significant dreams about some individual patients. These dreams may figure in the differential diagnosis of that person's ailment. For instance, a dream about a howling dog, hooting owl, or whistling bird may presage death.[2]

A number of associative symbols are generally well known throughout the South. One such association is light (good) and dark (evil). Mr. Lee told about the use of associative symbols in a dream about one client in which there was a dark shadow around the client indicating the man had been "rooted." Mr. Lee knew the man wanted to find out who had put the "fix" on him, but he could do nothing for him because it was outside his specialization of herbalism.

Some regional variants of the African American folk-medical system rely on *The Farmer's Almanac* and the use of the zodiac to "predict weather and regulate agricultural pursuits. They also affect the body, and their supposed effect on the human organism is the basis of a constant and lively practice of self-medication, dietary regulation and behavioral modification of various sorts" (Snow 1977:36).

Mr. Lee states that the moon affects health in general and that the astrological sign under which a person is born will determine characteristics of an individual; for example, will he/she be good or bad, tall or short? He feels the alignment of the moon and the stars at the time of his birth, October 31, 1910, is partly responsible for his own parapsychological abilities, which include clairvoyance and prophetic dreams. The sign also is believed to affect the monthly moods and dreams a person has. While Mr. Lee acknowledges some effects of the moon and astrological signs on humans, he does not refer to the astrological chart or almanac in making a diagnosis or in prescribing treatments.

Mr. Lee feels that the moon figures significantly in the life processes, for example, in planting, selection, and preparation of medical herbs for application. He states that the best medicine is prepared when the moon is full because it "tastes better and holds its strength better."

Mr. Lee experiences "flashes of insight." He finds these extremely difficult to describe or even to articulate. These insights enable him to "look into" a person and determine the nature of the problem. He has not been able to teach this skill. These insights are perceived to be a "gift from God."

Mr. Lee is an active member of the Mt. View A.M.E. Zion Church. His fellow church members come to him for medicine for arthritis, "ailing in the back," colds, indigestion, and so on. He feels that his ability to heal is an expression of his belief.

Mr. Lee's diagnoses, in keeping with a widespread Southern belief, include some symbolism; for example, in dreams a dark shadow warns of "rooting," and the howling dog and hooting owl presage death. Hand (1980) provides a fascinating collection of cross-cultural data on symbolism and magic in folk medicine. He examines such key elements as "the magical transfer of disease," "passing through," "physical harm," "sickness and death by conjury," and "over and out." Symbolism and magic in folk medicine are rejected in strict conventional medical diagnoses, and yet a certain consistency of observations of symptoms and prognosis of disease in folk medicine is often empirically valid.

In the modern community many resort to folk medicine but also turn to conventional medicine when they think it is more appropriate and if they can afford it. It is not uncommon for people to use both folk medicine and biomedicine concurrently.

NOTES

1. All quotes in the body of the text that do not have a citation are from Mr. Lee.

2. Such symbols as the owl as an ill omen are found throughout Africa and Europe and may be of either origin in this case.

Chapter 4

Classification of the Materia Medica and Illustrations

Mr. Lee's herbal pharmacopoeia is based mostly on the local botanical species found in Chatham and Lee counties in North Carolina. He also uses some species which are nonindigenous to the area, for example, *Aloe vera*. A detailed account of some of the medical botanicals used by Mr. Lee is given in Part Two.

The environment supports an extensive variety of plants. Chatham and Lee counties are located in the Piedmont on the eastern side of North Carolina. The rolling natural landscape extends across a variety of unconsolidated erosion materials: sand, red and yellow clays, flood plains, silts, and loams. The ecology is further diversified as it extends from the cooler deciduous forests of the North to the pines in the South.[1] This setting provides many types of natural botanical plants and enables Mr. Lee to collect numerous species of wild medicinal plants in addition to cultivating his own herb garden.[2]

Mr. Lee's botanical repertoire represents the combination of the three major cultures evident in this population. The majority of the herbs were known to the Cherokee and were and are used medicinally in a similar fashion.[3] Corresponding genera of African and New World botanicals were recognized by the slaves. They began experimenting and were able to make use of the New World herbs, which they then incorporated with their ethnopharmacopoeia.[4] Europeans introduced many of their own herbs and simples. Perhaps the best known introduced herb is *Plantago major* or plantain, known also as the Englishman's footprint.

CLASSIFICATION

The use of the herbs has been continuous. The people trust and appreciate them despite the development and influx of modern medicine. Mr. Lee has become skilled in the recognition and use of the botanicals. He has knowledge which spans this natural pharmacy from the search for wild specimens and cultivation of domesticated plants to the administration of medical plant therapy. Mr. Lee has categorized the botanicals according to a classification of his own. The four primary categories are (1) taste, (2) quantitative efficacy, (3) speed of response, and (4) toxicity.

The first quality, "taste," is best demonstrated by "strength." Mr. Lee illustrates this by contrasting the very strong acrid taste of poke root (*Phytolacca americana*) to the mild pleasurable taste of mint (*Mentha arvensis*). The amount of flavor or taste functions in direct relationship to the amount of the herb used.

The quantitative efficacy of the herb comprises (1) its age, (2) the amount used, and (3) the patient's physical response. First, the effect of the active ingredients varies with the "age" of the herb; the young plant, or part thereof, has little effect, while the mature plant has full power. A sample of a year-old poke root is not as powerful as that of a five-year-old root of poke root. Larger amounts of roots or leaves produce stronger medicine. Finally, a potent herb brings about an immediate response and the person "can feel it working on the problem." For example, Mr. Lee classifies grip grass (*Sisyrinchium*) as a potent herb which produces a strong reaction. Catnip (*Nepeta cataria*) has only a medium reaction.

An estimate of the comparative effectiveness is demonstrated in the contrast between an active herb, such as rabbit tobacco (*Gnaphalium obtusioflium*), which "stimulates a person right away," and plantain (*Plantago major*), a mildly active herb, which has a slow reaction.

A toxic herb is classified as a "powerful" herb. It may be either a well-known poisonous herb, such as nightshade (*Solanium niqrum*), or an herb such as jimsonweed (*Datura stramonium*), which has harmful side effects if ingested or smoked and inhaled. Taken improperly, powerful herbal remedies may be harmful.

The selection and preparation of the herbs are affected by various factors. The active ingredients contained in a plant change with the seasons of the year. For example, sap is believed to be "settled" in the winter; this makes the root of a plant or the lower bark on a tree more potent. In the spring the sap rises, and, therefore, the upper sections of plants and trees are more vigorous.

The distribution of particular potency within plants depends not only on seasonal changes but on directional location. For example, bark is stripped from the north side of the tree because this side is not as directly exposed to the sun. It is believed that the sun may diminish the inherent strength in plants and trees. In harvesting the bark, Mr. Lee makes small downward strokes with a sharp axe. He collects from cherry and oak trees whether dead or alive. This practice differs from the associational methods described by Puckett. According to Puckett's sources (white informants from Ohio), upward strokes are used to collect the barks for emetics and downward strokes for laxative medicines (1980).

In the spring, the bark changes as the sap rises and is taken from the north side of the tree. In the winter, the sap settles in the bottom so Mr. Lee strips the bark from the bottom of the tree. The same seasonal forces affect the leaves and roots, so when they are gathered they are dried in the shade to preserve their effectiveness. However, a fresh plant has a higher chemical potency. For example, fresh pine top (*Pinus strobus*) and red oak bark (*Quercus rubra*) are more potent fresh than dry.

Odor is considered a significant characteristic in plant selection. Mr. Lee explains, "If it [herb] does not smell as I think it should, then I don't use it." Roots that have a sharp, pungent, or "bitter" odor are generally to be avoided. The smell is distinguished from taste; "most herbs have a bitter taste but they smell all right."

Mr. Lee's perceptions of "smell" and "taste" are remarkably consistent. Individual empirical categories of efficacy and use are difficult to measure with precision. He takes into consideration such factors as the age of a plant and believes that the biochemical virtues change with degree of growth, length and thickness of roots, and variations in the parts of the plants. He observes the immediate environment of the individual plant and assesses the amount of sun it receives.

ILLUSTRATIONS

Most of Mr. Lee's materia medica are part of the general folklore, as are their applications.[5] He has, however, some individual practices in his combination of specific herbs and in his methods of their preparation and administration for specific cures.

One example of this is combining equal portions of burdock (*Arctium minus*), dandelion (*Taraxacum officinale*), and white oak bark (*Quercus alba*) in a tea for varicose veins. A second example is mixing equal portions of catnip (*Nepeta cataria*), wild comfrey (*Cynoglossum virqinianum*), and the roots of black cohosh (*Cimicifuga racemosa*) in a tea to treat seizures. Another example is a treatment for diabetes and arthritis. The roots of sarsaparilla (*Menispermum canadense*) and black cohosh (*Cimicifuga racemosa*) are combined in corn whiskey or boiled in water and kept in the refrigerator. Bear's foot (*Polymnia uvedalia*) may be added if the affliction is severe. Perhaps the most potent herb in Mr. Lee's pharmacopoeia is the "powerful" poke root (*Phytolacca americana*). He recognizes its strength and discusses the caution needed in collecting the root. "This time of year [spring] is a good time to gather this poke root. In the wintertime you are not supposed to bother it, because it goes to sleep. Most all the herbs go to sleep a certain time of the year and it's more poisonous when they go to sleep. . . . But after they sit there and all of the sap goes right down in the roots, they get stronger and stronger."

Hattie Mae Lee described her own experience with poke root and its effectiveness as a medicinal herb for choking spasms in the throat.

> Now I have taken some. I began to get a choking here [throat], and it bothered me even if I drank water. I would hurt in there. So I knew about the poke root being good for your throat and things like that, so I decided to fix some. So I took mine at night. After I had only taken five doses, I haven't been bothered by it anymore.

A second example from the family history involves one of their daughters, who lives in New York City. She had a problem with cysts in the breasts. After repeated visits to physicians to have the cysts drained, she turned to her father's knowledge of herbs for additional help. A preparation of poke root was used and within a week the cysts disappeared.

John and Hattie Mae also tell about the use of poke root by the "old folks" for the "seven year itch."

> The seven year itch would break out on you. You just scratch, scratch, scratch. And the old folks would just bathe you in it [poke root]. It would kill that germ or whatever it was in your skin. Some of the children's feet were just gettin' raw from where they had been scratching. It was terrible. . . . You bathe in it [poke root solution] twice a day . . . and by the third day it's gone. But I'll tell you one thing; when they had it too strong [the solution], somebody had to hold you because it would burn you so bad. Usually it was when the skin was broken. . . . You have to be careful about how you use it.

In another case, a patient from Maryland told the author of his experience with a keloid at the top of his sternum. From time to time this scar would become irritated and infected. He applied a salve made of poke root (*Phytolacca americana*) and petroleum jelly and soon the keloid was gone.

Mr. Lee believes impurities or germs enter the blood system by "eating, drinking, using or touching unclean things, or by being unclean oneself." Impurities may be eliminated by using a blood purifier such as golden seal (*Hydrastis candensis*) or ginseng (*Panax quinquefolium*). These teas carry the impurities out of the system through perspiration, urine, and "body wastes." Pine top (*Pinus strobus*) tea is used for colds, as it "causes a certain amount of water to come out of the blood, because the blood becomes hot, resulting in perspiration, which eliminates the impurities from the blood."

Four other examples of dealing with impurities are given in the treatment of three ear infections and a skin rash. First, Mr. Lee recounts the story of a young boy:

> There is a young boy who came up here . . . and he went fishing with us. My son and I were down there at the river and he came down

Classification of the Materia Medica

where we were fishing. He had talked with us about his ear bothering him. He decided he would try some of this sarsaparilla. . . . He and my son chewed some that day that we were down fishing. He took some with him and about a week or so later, he came back up and was talking with us about how his ear had stopped running.

Hattie Mae, herself, provided a second example. She had been out of town and when she returned she found one of her daughters had an ear infection.

> My daughter had an earache and it wouldn't drain out. Now it went down into her gland and it formed a little pottage egg on the side of her neck. . . . I carried her to the doctor and he said it was some earache that wouldn't drain out. So he gave me some pills for her and he told me that if they didn't move it, to bring her back and he would lance it. So I gave her this medicine and it didn't move. So I started giving her sarsaparilla. I just boiled the root, and I gave it to her, and it moved it.

A local patient of the Lees told the author how she had been helped by the Lees when she had a problem with neck pains and fluid and wax buildup in her ears. She had gone to the local physician several times but had found no relief. She then consulted Mr. Lee. He prepared a medicine using black cohosh (*Cimicifuga racemosa*) and sarsaparilla (*Menispermum canadense*). She took the medicine three times a day and within a few days the problem began to clear up.

The fourth example was given by Hattie Mae Lee.

> There was a girl who worked in _____ who came down here and she had a rash on her. She said it itched her so bad. And Lee got some nightshade and told her to rub it on her. She rubbed it on her, and she said it just stopped the itching. She wasn't bothered by it anymore.

Lee's practice extends beyond physiological troubles such as infection and "impurities." He also treats "natural" injuries. For example, Hattie Mae tells about an electrician who came to them for help after severely burning his hand.

> There was an electrician who came here. He had been to the hospital. Somehow he had caught a hot wire and it had ruined his hand. He had to go to the hospital with it. He said that they had doctored on it, but his 'liders' were drawn, and his hand just felt numb. He couldn't use it like he had been. He asked us if we could do something. I said, "Well, I believe that aloe would help you." I said, "Lee, get him some aloe." Lee went out there and got some and gave him some pieces, and he rubbed it all on his hand. And he talked for a while and then he said, "It seems like my 'liders' are beginning to feel more limber." He could move his hand much easier when he left.

A relative of the author's who was visiting from Illinois went to Mr. Lee's on one of the field trips. She had severe arthritis and suffered considerable pain. She walked with a cane. Mr. Lee gave her some sarsaparilla (*Menispermum canadense*), black cohosh (*Cimicifuga racemosa*), and bear's foot (*Polymnia uvedalia*). After taking several doses she felt improvement and reduced pain. She was able to walk without her cane.

A second example of the effectiveness of sarsaparilla (*Menispermum canadense*) and black cohosh (*Cimicifuga racemosa*) was observed in the case of a vendor in Washington, D.C., on Howard University's campus. He is constantly exposed to the elements in all weather. Cold and dampness brought on acute attacks of his arthritis. He began taking Mr. Lee's medicine (sarsaparilla and black cohosh) on a regular basis. The effect has been a reduction in pain. The previous limits on his movements have been noticeably lessened.

Several students over the years who have come into the author's office have told of their own personal experiences with Mr. Lee. Recently one student said, "I have trouble with asthma. My mom had taken me to the doctors but their medicine didn't work. She went to Mr. Lee and got some medicine and it worked. Now, whenever I get an attack, she just goes straight to him."

Lee's therapy also includes a number of nonbotanical remedies (see Appendix). The use of cobwebs is known all over the world as a natural dressing in first aid comparable to an adhesive bandage.[6] Mr. Lee uses a combination of cobweb in a mixture with dirt dauber (wasp) nest and soot. Hattie Mae tells of a time Mr. Lee used this combination to treat a cut that would not stop bleeding.

> One of my children got hurt real bad on her knee and it was bleeding so bad. My husband got some dirt dauber nest . . . and some spider web and soot, and he put that on the cut, and then he bandaged it up and it stopped the bleeding. The child's leg got all right and there wasn't even a black streak where the cut was. It cleared up and it held together good.

Mr. Lee's collection, selection, and preparation of the herbs used as materia medica essentially reflect the "folk wisdom and mother wit" that have been passed down from antiquity to the present generation. This book about Mr. John Lee has presented a picture of an herbal healer, who practices a regional variant of the African American folk medical system.

NOTES

1. See Braun (1964).
2. Identification and classification of the herbs used by Mr. Lee were made by Dr. James A. Duke, Chief of Economic Botany of the United States

Department of Agriculture. Collected samples are in the Howard University Department of Sociology/Anthropology.

3. See Mooney (1932), Angier (1978), and Hamel and Chiltoskey (1975). There are general resemblances among differing species of herbs found in various parts of the world which have similar chemical properties, for example, pennyroyal (*Pycnanthus*). The American Indians were quite familiar with the uses of pennyroyal tea and the colonists in the South and Pennsylvania also recognized it. Pennyroyal was known to the Africans. In this instance the same genera, albeit different species, are used for the same purpose. Also in terms of major culture areas from moderate through tropical zones, marijuana (*Cannabis sativa*) is universal (including the desert areas) and generally recognized for its healing properties as well as its hallucinogenic characteristics.

4. Ayensu (1978); Hutchinson and Dalziel (1936); Watt and Breyer-Brandwijk (1962).

5. Porcher (1863); Krochmal et al. (1969); Morton (1974); Krochmal and Krochmal (1975).

6. Cobwebs probably have an antifibrinolytic activity which is directly antagonistic to the breakdown of clots (personal communication from Dr. Harvey Klein, Chief of the Department of Transfusion Medicine, National Institutes of Health, Bethesda, Maryland).

Part Two

Herbal Repertoire

Mr. Lee knows over a hundred medicinal herbs. A few of these he very rarely uses. Sixty herbs he works with most frequently are listed here, arranged alphabetically by scientific nomenclature. Scientific names are followed by verncular names, which are the ones used by Mr. Lee. His classification of herbs is included. The information is reduced to a set of symbols as follows:

T = taste	S = strong
R = reaction	M = medium or mild
A = active	Powerful = poisonous or harmful
V = very	____ = unclassified

The use of the herb is described. Finally, a list of the main active ingredients of each herb is provided whenever possible.

Various references were consulted:

James Duke, *C.R.C. Handbook of Medicinal Herbs* (1985), (henceforth, Duke); and J. Duke, *Father Nature's Farmacy,* computer data base (1990) (henceforth, *FNF)*

A. Krochmal and C. Krochmal, *A Guide to Medicinal Plants of the United States* (1975)

P. H. List and L. Horhammer (eds.), *Hagers Handbuch der Pharmazeutischen Praxis* (1969-1979) (henceforth, *Hagers*)[1]

J. Morton, *Major Medicinal Plants: Botany, Culture and Uses* (1975)

W. C. Sturtevant, *The Wealth of India: A Dictionary of Indian Raw Materials and Industrial Products* (1963) (henceforth, *Wealth of Ind*)

J. M. Watt and M. G. Breyer-Brandwijk, *The Medicinal and Poisonous Plants of Southern and Eastern Africa* (1962)

H. Felter and J. Lloyd, *King's American Dispensatory* (1983) (henceforth, Felter and Lloyd).

SCIENTIFIC NAME: Acorus calamus

LOCAL NAME: Flagroot (Sweet Flag)

LEE'S CLASSIFICATION: ST SR A

USE(S): Gas, indigestion, heartburn, colic, upset stomach, menstrual cramps, ulcers, worms

ACTIVE INGREDIENTS:
Acolamone, acoragermacrone, acoric acid, acorone, acoroxide, asaraldehyde, asarone, beta-asarone, azulene, calamente, calameone, calamenol, calamenone, calamol, camphene, camphor, choline, cineole, dextrin, dextrose, dimethylamine, eugenol, n-heptylic acid, isoacolamone, isoacorone, linalool, methylamine, methyl-eugenol, palmitic acid, parasarone, pinene, and trimethylamine. (Duke: 14-15; *FNF:* 12-14)

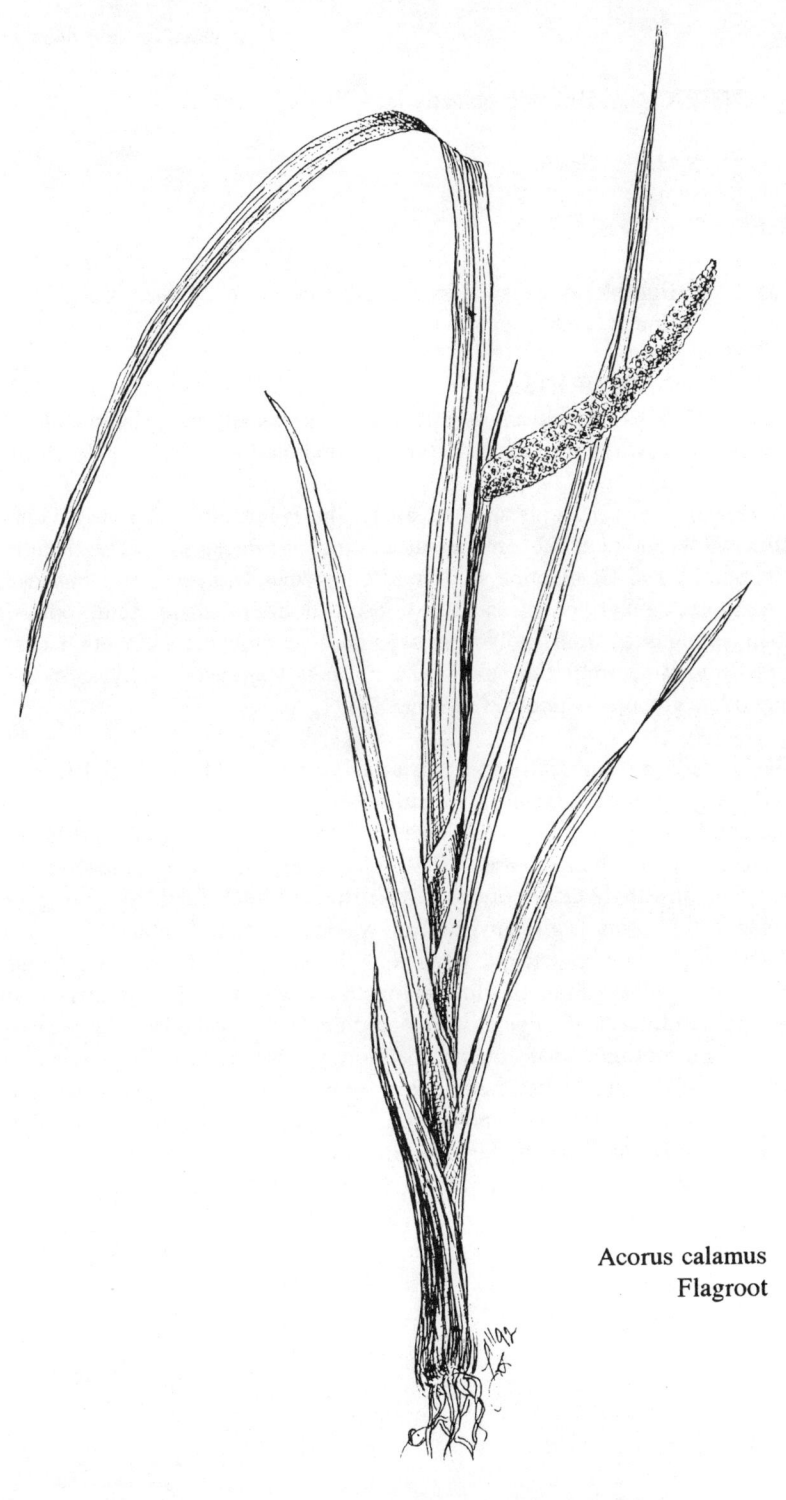

Acorus calamus
Flagroot

SCIENTIFIC NAME: Allium sativum

LOCAL NAME: Garlic

LEE'S CLASSIFICATION: ST VSR A

USE(S): High blood pressure, colds, sore throat, cough, consumption, liver ailment, emphysema

ACTIVE INGREDIENTS:
Bulbs on distillation yield an essential oil containing allylpropyl-disulfide, diallyl disulfide and two more sulfur-containing compounds. (*Wealth of Ind.*: 59)

Mono-, di-, tri-, and polysulfides, alliin; the lyoenzyme alliinase divides into alliin and its antibacterial components allicine, pyroraceuric acid, and ammonia. Vitamins A and C, nicotine acid amide, enzymes (i.e., alliinase, myrosinase, peroxidose, deoxyribonuclease, tyrosinose), choline, rhodanic acid, iodine, very small amounts of uran, polyoses, saponines, carbohydrates, methyl cysteine, methyl cystisine, sulfoxide, allyl cysteine; beta-L-glutanyl-s-allyl-cysteine, and nine other glutamylpeptides. (*Hagers:* 1211)

Alanine, allicin, alliin, alliinase, allistatin-1, allistatin-11, (-)-S-allyl-L-cysteine, allyl-methyl-sulfide, allyl-propyl-disulfide, arginine, ascorbic acid, aspartic acid, calcium, carbohydrates, beta-carotene, choline, chromium, citral, cobalt, copper, cystine, desoxyribonuc-lease, diallyl-disulfide, diallyl-trisulfide, dimethyl-disulfide, dimethyl-sulfide, dimehtyl-trisulfide, EO, fat, fiber, foliacin, geraniol, glutamic acid, beta-L-glutamyl-S-allyl-cysteine, gamma-L-glutamyl-isoleucine, gamma-L-glutamyl-L-leucine, gamma-L-glutamyl-L-phenylalanine, gamma-L-glutamyl-L-valine,gamma-L-glutamyl-methionine,gamma-L-glutamyl-S-methyl-L-cysteinesulfoxide, glycine, histidine, iodine, iron, isoleucine, leucine, linalool, lysine, magnesium, manganese, methionine, S-methyl-L-cysteine-sulfoxide, myrosinase, niacin, nickel, peroxidase, alpha-phellandrene, beta-phellandrene, phenylalanine, phosphorus, potassium, proline, protein, riboflavin, saponin, scorodin-A, serine, sodium, thiamin, threonine, 2,3,4-trithiapentane, tryptophan, tyrosine, tyrosinase, uranium, valine, water, zinc. (*FNF:* 22-25)

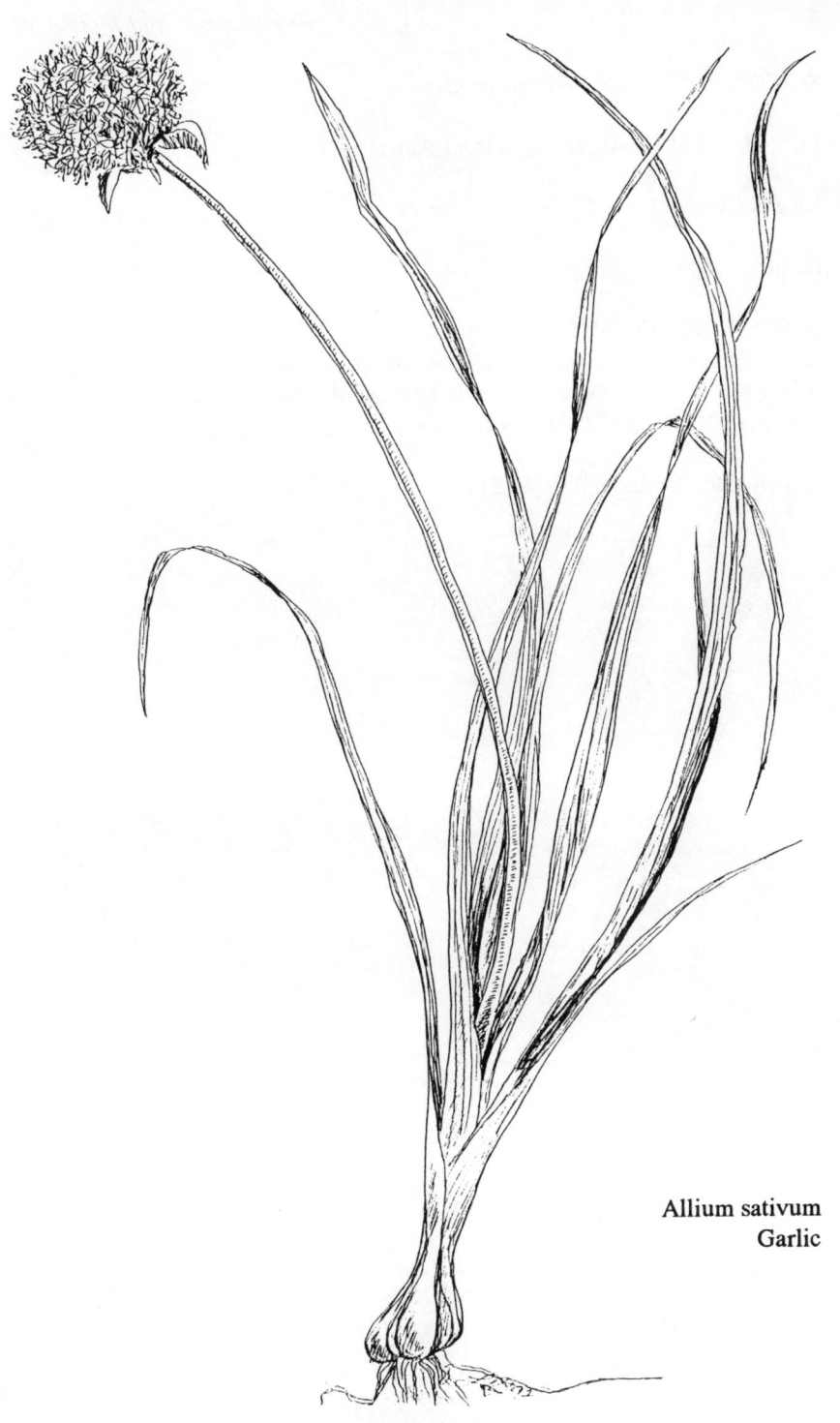

Allium sativum
Garlic

SCIENTIFIC NAME: Alnus serrulata

LOCAL NAME: Alder Tag (Hazel Alder)

LEE'S CLASSIFICATION: ___ SR A

USE(S): Fly Repellent

ACTIVE INGREDIENTS:
Bark: tannin, oils, resin; Leaves: tannin, oils, resin but in a lesser quantity (other species of alnus contain ellagotannins of interest to the National Cancer Institute). (Felter and Lloyd: Vol. I 147)

Hyperoside, tannin. (*FNF:* 25-26)

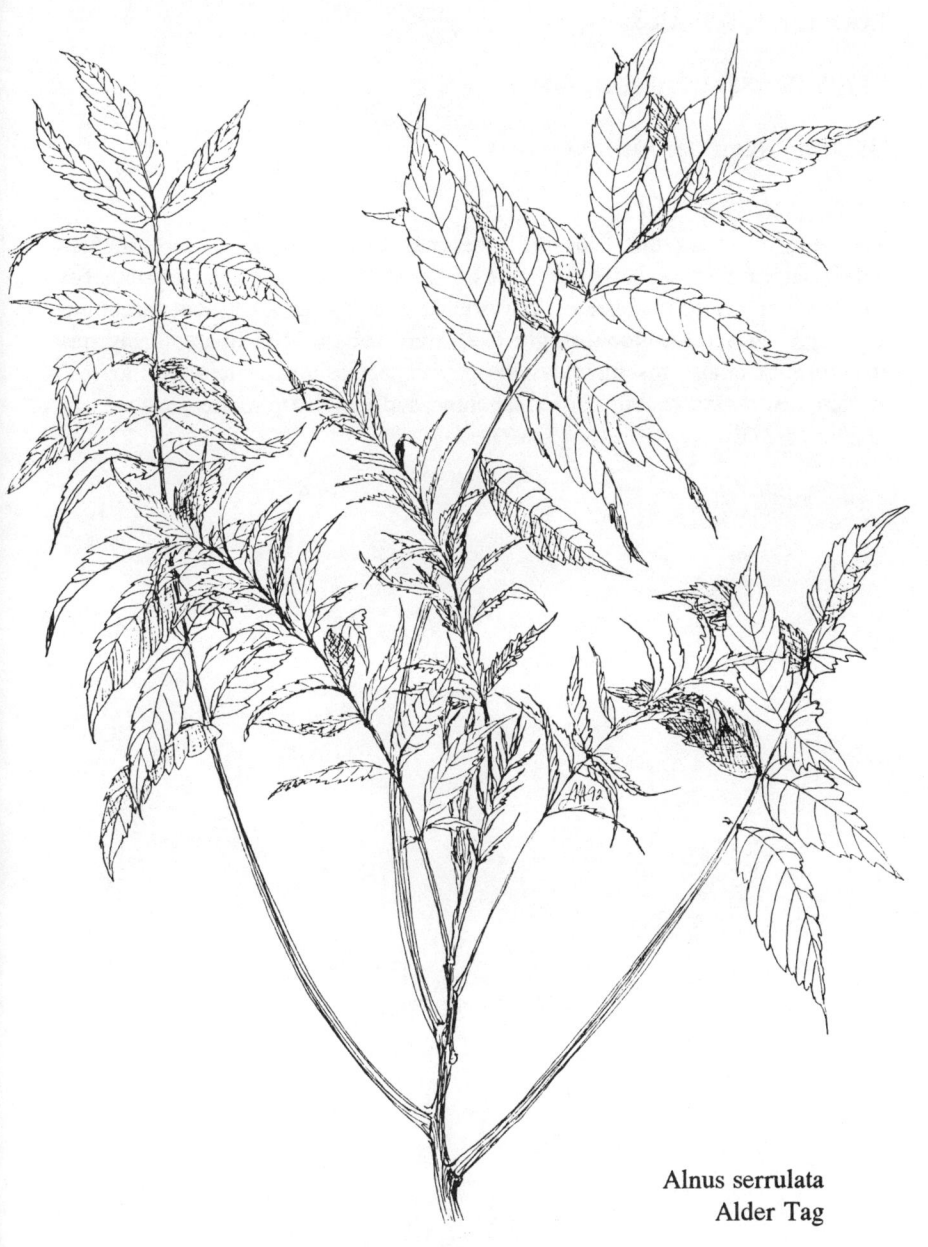

Alnus serrulata
Alder Tag

SCIENTIFIC NAME: Aloe vera

LOCAL NAME: Aloe

LEE'S CLASSIFICATION: MT SR VA

USE(S): Burns, stomach troubles

ACTIVE INGREDIENTS:
Albumin, aloe-emodin, aloesin, aloesone, aloetic acid, aloins, amylase, anthracene, arabinose, barbaloin, beta-barbaloin, calcium, calcium-oxalate, beta-carotene, chloride, cholesterol, chrysophanic acid, cinnamic acid, creatinine, folic acid, galactose, globulin, glucose, iron, isobarbaloin, lipase, manganese, mannose, mucilage, niacinamide, phosphorus, potassium, protein, purine, resin, resitannols, rhamnose, riboflavin, saponins, sodium, thiamin, urea, xylose, zinc.
(*FNF:* 26-27)

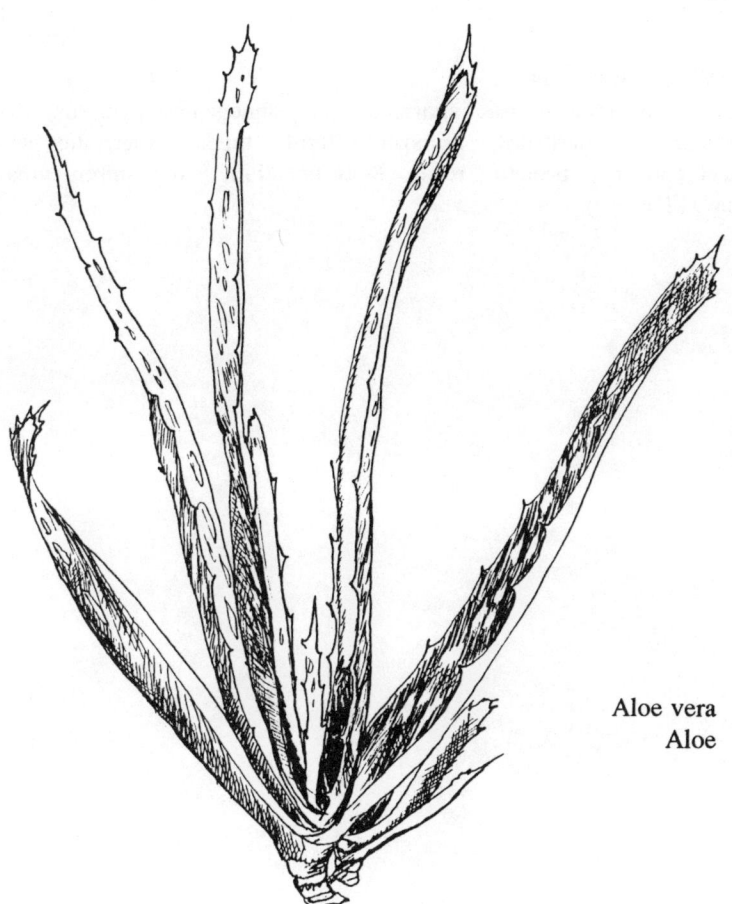

Aloe vera
Aloe

SCIENTIFIC NAME: Apocynum cannabinum

LOCAL NAME: Gall-of-the-Earth

LEE'S CLASSIFICATION: St SR A

USE(S): Stomach problems, urinary tract problems, blood purifier, arthritis, sores

ACTIVE INGREDIENTS:
Alpha-amyrin, androsterol, apocannoside, cannogenin, cymarin, cymarol, cynocannoside, harmalol, homoandrosterol, lupeol, oleanolic acid, p-oxyacetophenone, protein, resin, k-strophanthin, strophanthin-cymaroside, tannin. (FNF: 59)

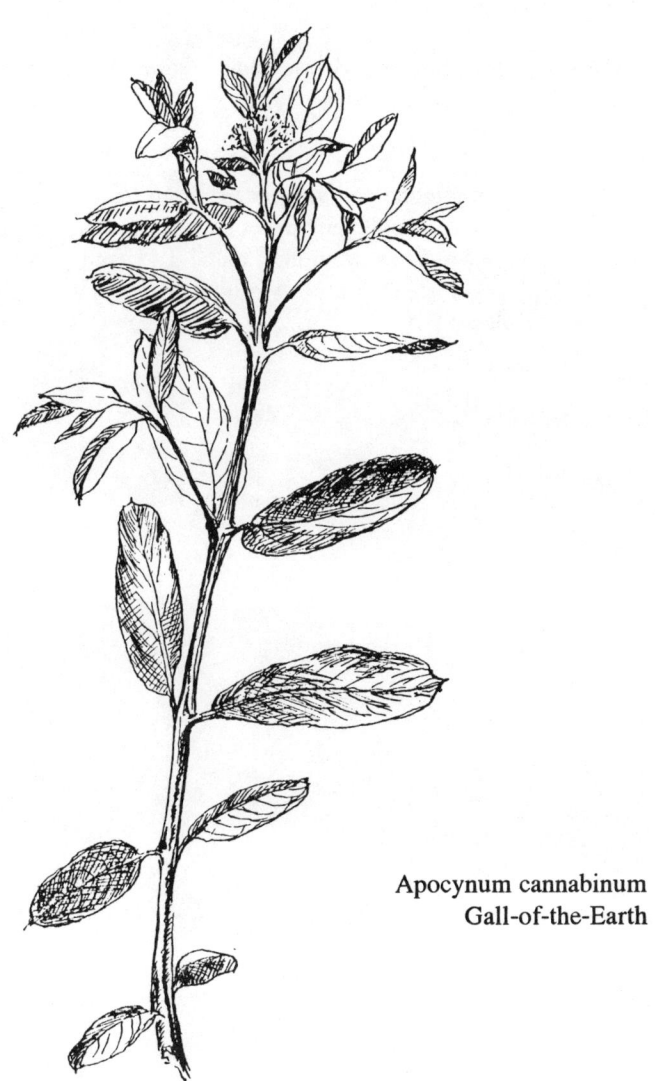

Apocynum cannabinum
Gall-of-the-Earth

SCIENTIFIC NAME: Arctium minus

LOCAL NAME: Burdock

LEE'S CLASSIFICATION: MT MR MA

USE(S): Sores, swelling, coughs, colds, canker sores, gout, rheumatism, varicose veins, stomach trouble

ACTIVE INGREDIENTS:
Leaves: arctiol, dehydrofukinone, eremophilene, beta- eudesmol, fukinone, fukinanolide, and taraxasterol; Roots: polyphenolic acids (caffeic, chlorogenic), gamma-guanidimo-n-isovaleric and propionic, arctic acid, and polyacetylenes; Seeds: glucoside arctiin, chlorogenic acid, two lignans (lappaol A and B), and a germacranolide. (Duke: 54)

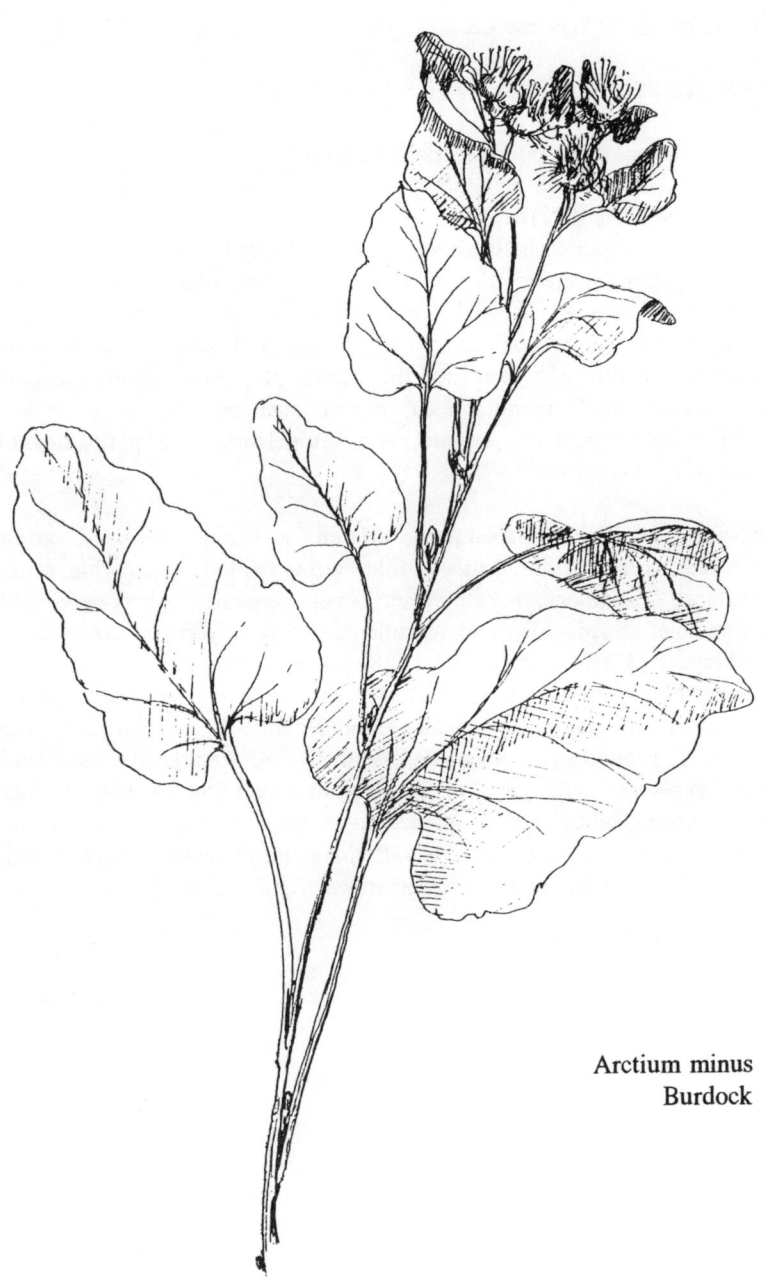

Arctium minus
Burdock

SCIENTIFIC NAME: Artemisia absinthium

LOCAL NAME: Wormwood

LEE'S CLASSIFICATION: VST SR VA Powerful

USE(S): Indigestion, poor blood circulation

ACTIVE INGREDIENTS:
Essential oil contains phellandrene, pinene, thujone (3 to 12 percent), thijul alcohol, thujyl, acetate, thujyl isovalerate, bisabolene, thujyl palmitate, camphene, cadinene, nerol and azulene (chamazulene,3,6,-dihydrochamazulene,5,6,-dihydrochamazulene), formic and salicyclic acids are in the saponifications lyes of wormwood oil. Bitter glucosides, absinthin, absinthic acid, succinic acid, tannin, resin, starch, malates, nitrates of potassium. Lactones include arabsin, artabin, and ketopelenolide (a germacroanolide). (Duke: 67)

Artabasin, achillicin, anabisinthin, artabin, artenisetin, arabsin, artemetin, arthamarin, arthamarinin, arthamaridin, arthamaridinine, ascorbic acid, ash, bisabolene, cadinene, campnene, beta-carotene, beta-caryophyllene, chamazulene, 3,6,-dihydrochamazulene, 5,6-dihydrochamazuelen, 3,7-dioxabicycl- (3,3,0)-octane, EO, CIS-epoxyocimene, trans- epoxyocimene, formic-acid, 5-hydroxy-3,6,7.3',4'-penta-methoxyflavone, inulobiose, isorhamnetin-3-0-rhamno-glucoside, ketopelenolide-A, nicotinic acid, palmitic acid, fat, patuletin-3-0-glucoside, patuletin-3-0-rhamnoside, phellandrene, pinene, pipecolic acid, protein, quebrachitol, quercitin-3-0-beta-D-glucoside, rutin, sabinene, salicylic acid, spinacetin-3-0-glucoside, spinacetin-3-0-rhamnoglucoside, tannin, alpha-thujone, beta-thujone, thujyl-alcohol, thujyl-isovalerate, thujyl-palmitate, trans-dehydromatricaria-ester. (*FNF:* 64-5)

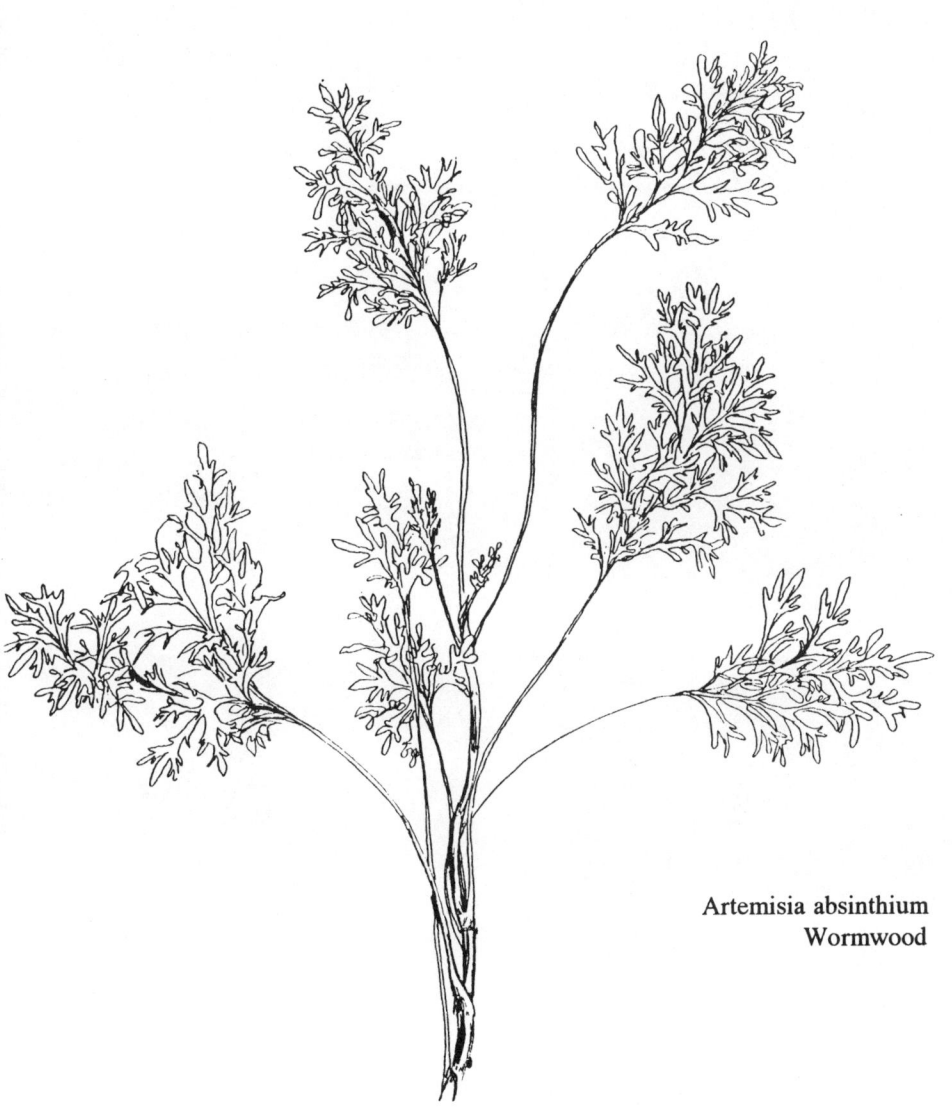

Artemisia absinthium
Wormwood

SCIENTIFIC NAME: Asarum virginicum

LOCAL NAME: Heart Leaf

LEE'S CLASSIFICATION: ___ MR A

USE(S): Hairdressing, dandruff

ACTIVE INGREDIENTS:
Aristolic acid. (Duke personal communication)

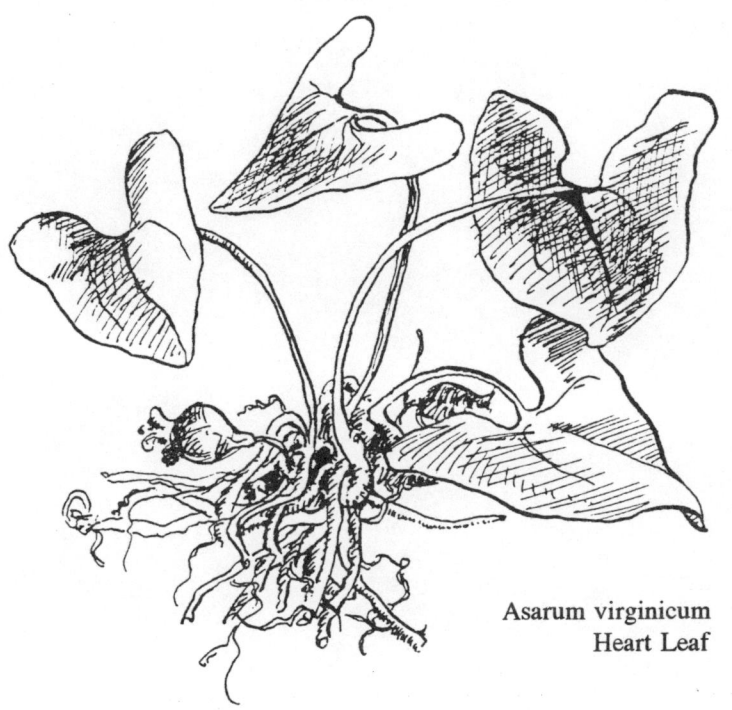
Asarum virginicum
Heart Leaf

SCIENTIFIC NAME: Asclepias spp.

LOCAL NAME: Milkweed

LEE'S CLASSIFICATION: ___ SR A

USE(S): Sores, insect bites, wasp stings, poison oak, poison ivy, bleeding cuts

ACTIVE INGREDIENTS:
Latex: caoutchouc, digitalis-like mixture of alpha- and beta-asclepiadin, antitumor beta-sitosterol and alpha- and beta-amyrin, and its acetate dextros and wax. (Duke: 72)

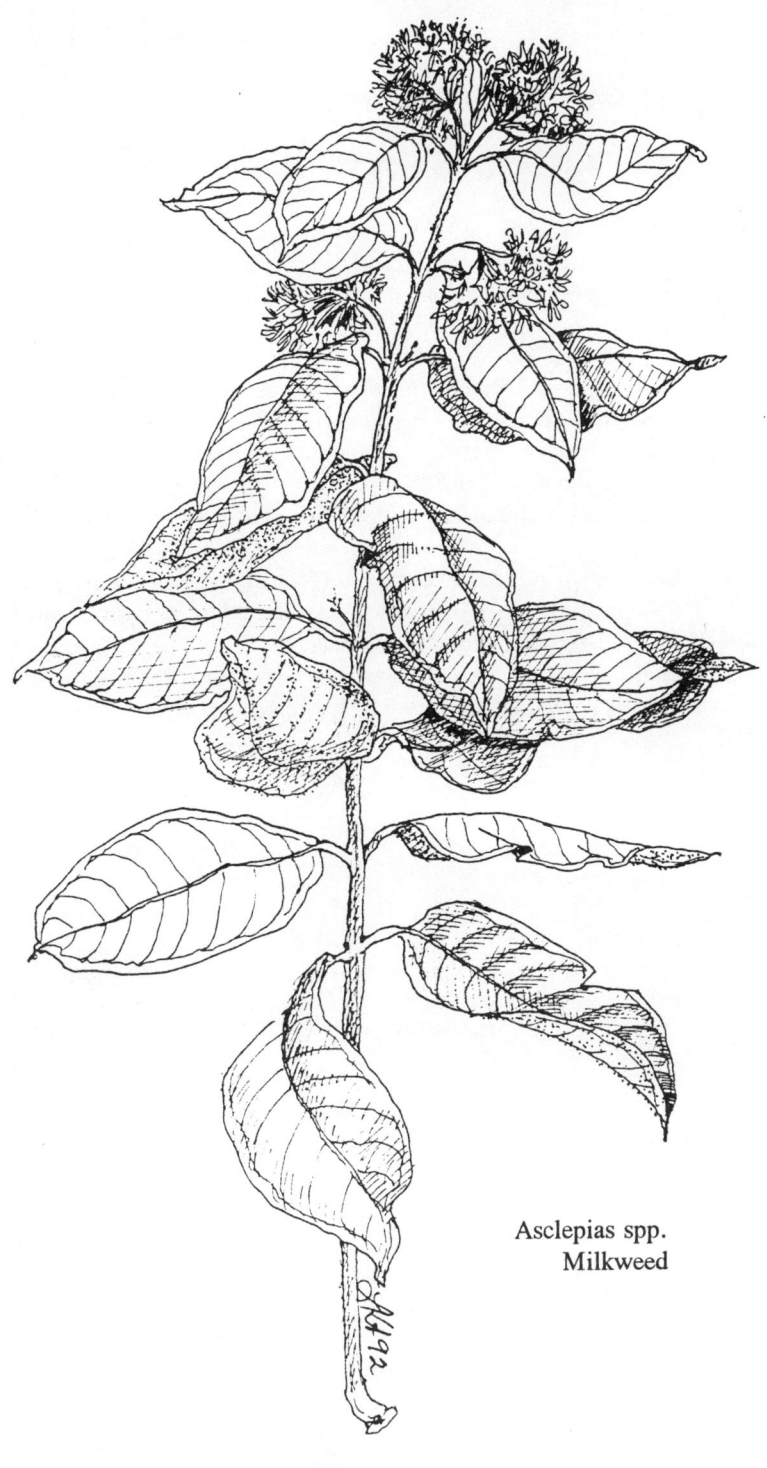

Asclepias spp.
Milkweed

SCIENTIFIC NAME: Baptisia tinctoria

LOCAL NAME: Wild Indigo

LEE'S CLASSIFICATION: MT SR A

USE(S): Swelling, bruises, spider bites, insect bites, and diabetes

ACTIVE INGREDIENTS:
Stem and leaves: alkaloids cytisine (baptitoxine, sophorine, laburnine, ulexine), methyl cystisine, (caulophylline), anagyrine (monolupine, rhombinine), and 13-hydroxysparteine; Leaves: baptisol, luteolin, luteolin-7-0-rhamnnoglucoside, orobol, orobol-7-0-rhamnoglucoside, pseudobaptigenin, pseudobaptgenin-7-0-rhamnoglucoside, scopoletin and scopoletin-7-0-glucoside. (*Hagers:* 355-56)

Anagyrine, baptisine, baptisol, biochanin-A, biochanin-A-7-0-rhamnoglucoside, cytisine, genistein, genistein-7-0-rhamnoglucoside, gum, 13-hydroxysparteine, luteolin, luteolin-7-0-rhamnoglucoside, methyl-cytisine, orobol, orobol-7-0-rhamnoglucoside, pseudobaptigenin, pseudo-baptigenin-7-0-rhamnoglucoside, resin, scopoletin, scopoletin-7-0-glucoside, sparteine, tectorigenin. (*FNF:* 90-91)

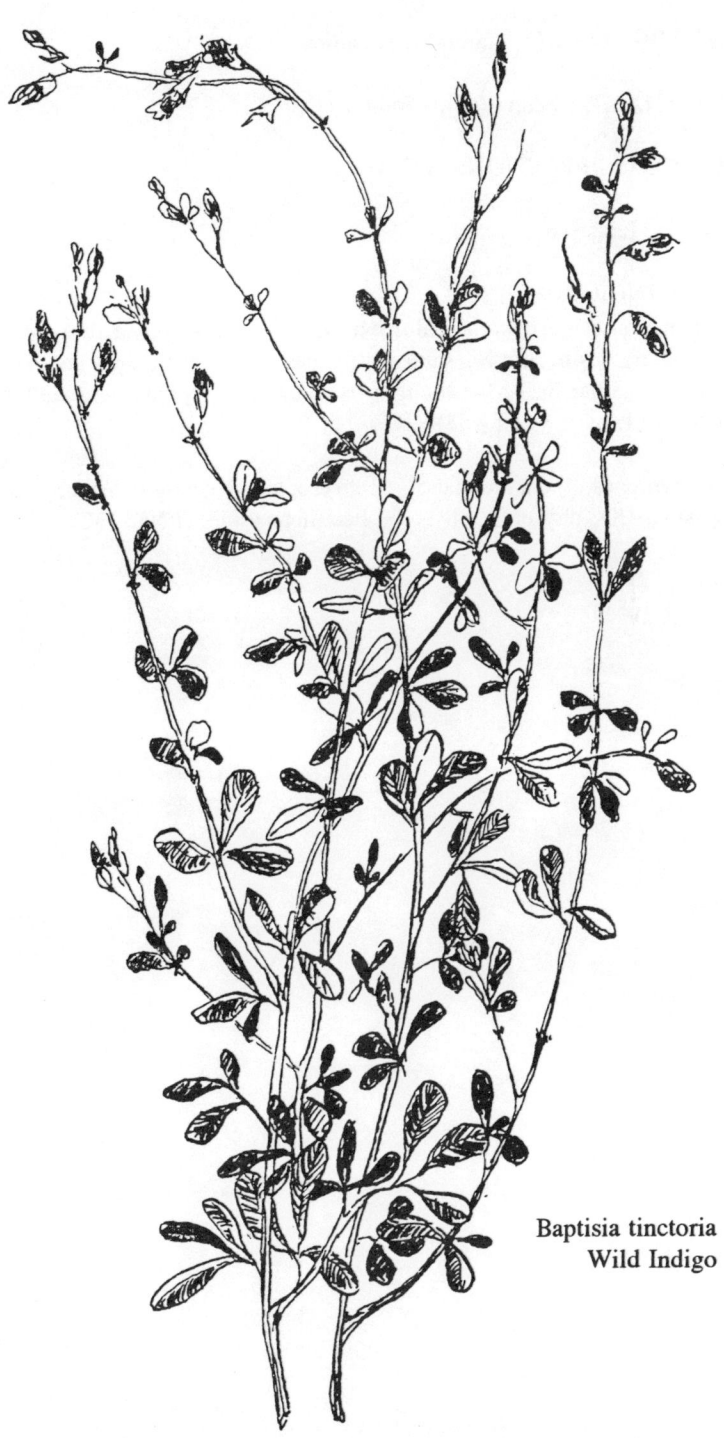
Baptisia tinctoria
Wild Indigo

SCIENTIFIC NAME: Cassia marilandica

LOCAL NAME: Senna (Wild Senna)

LEE'S CLASSIFICATION: MT MR A

USE(S): Laxative

ACTIVE INGREDIENTS:
Albumen, mucilage, starch, chlorophyll, yellow coloring matter, volatile oil, fatty matter, resin, lignin, salts of potassium and calcium, and a principle resembling cathartin. Also thought to contain chrysophan and cathartic acid. (Felter and Lloyd: Vol 1 458)

Anthraquinones, chrysophanol, chrysophanol-beta-glucoside, 2-emodin-heteroside, EO, physcion, physcion-beta-heteroside. (*FNF:* 132)

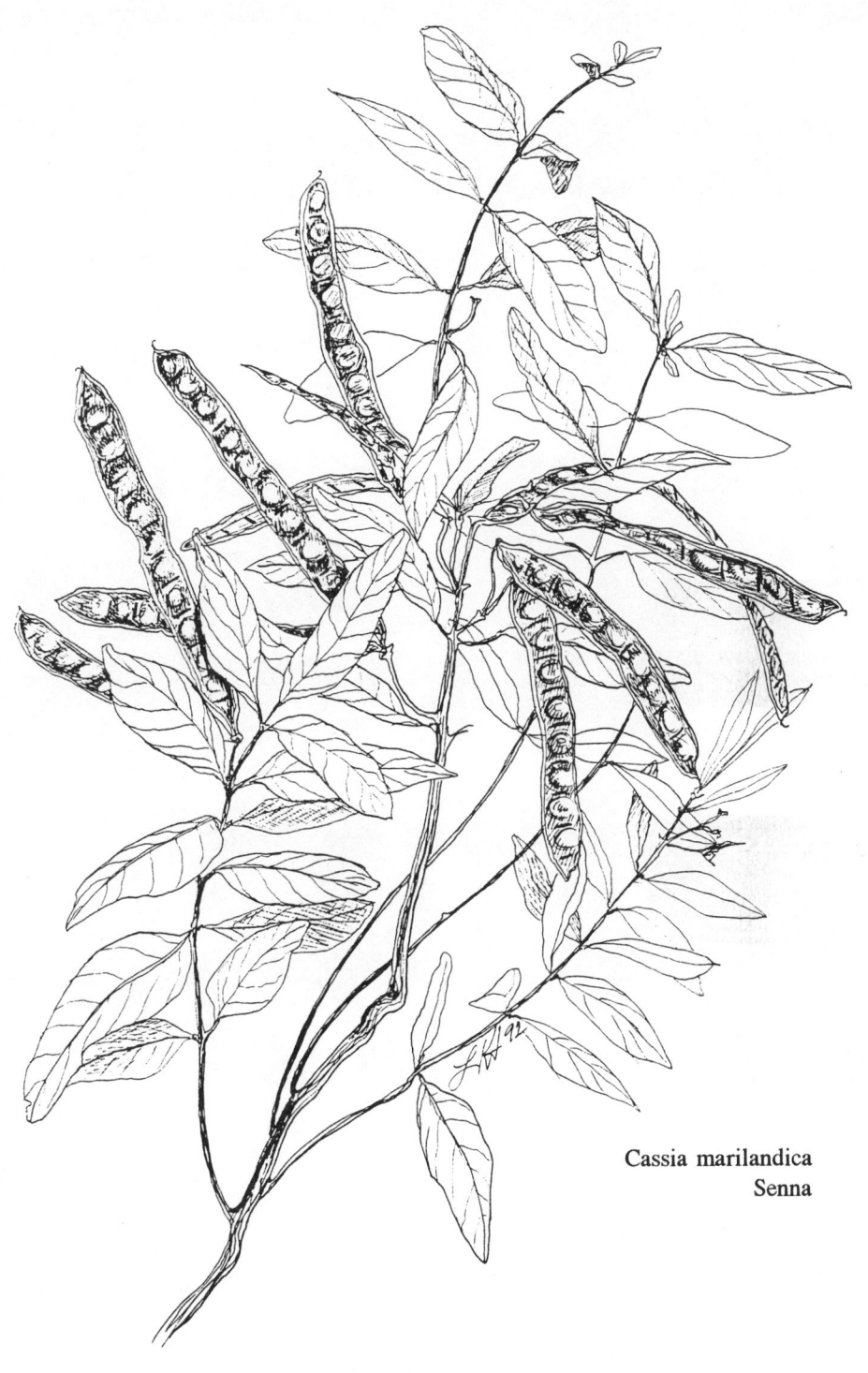

Cassia marilandica
Senna

SCIENTIFIC NAME: Chenopodium sp?

LOCAL NAME: Fly Weed

LEE'S CLASSIFICATION: ___ SR VA Powerful

USE(S): Kills flies

ACTIVE INGREDIENTS:
Essential oil: oleum chenopodil. (Felter and Lloyd: 494-95)

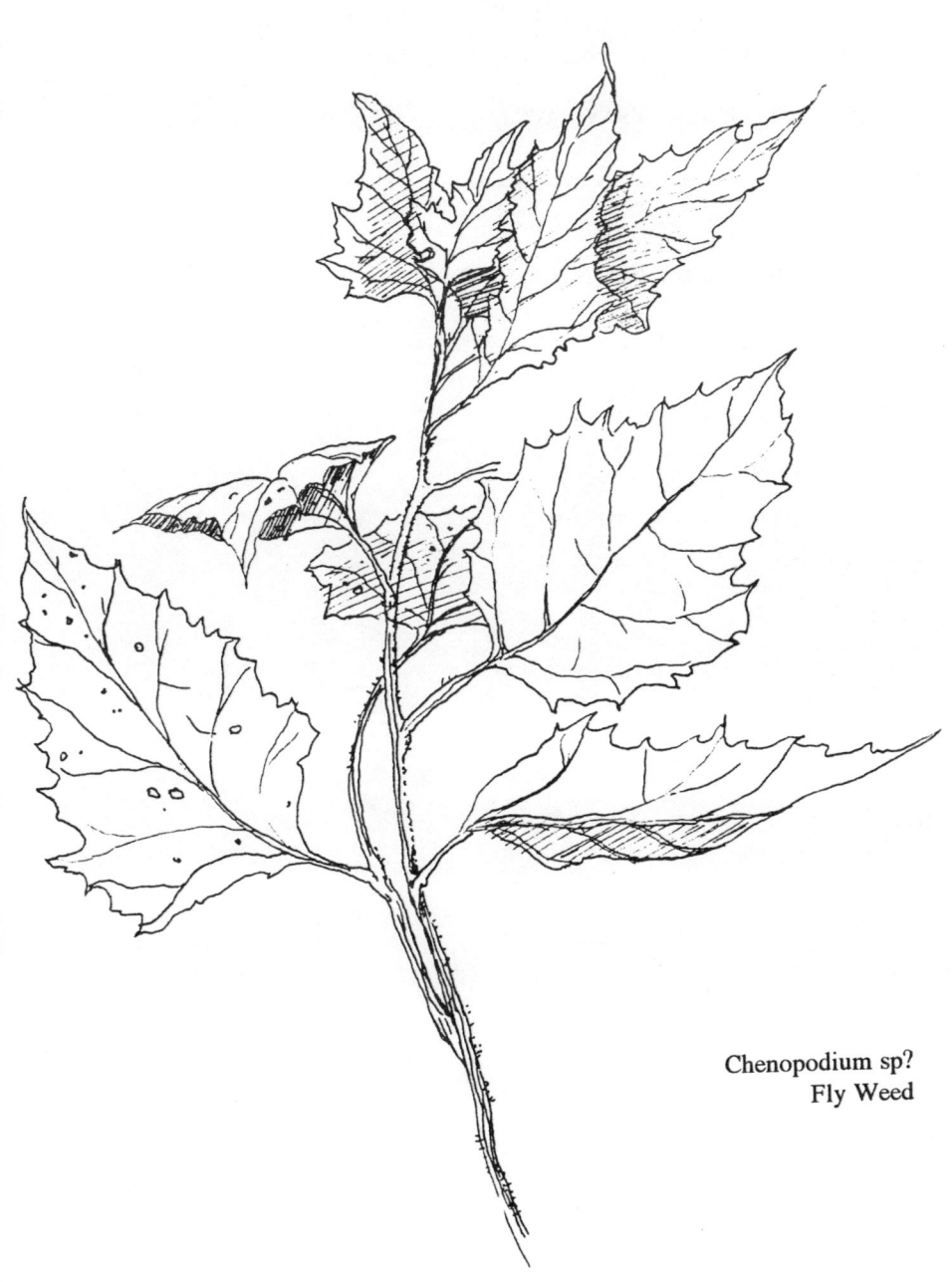

Chenopodium sp?
Fly Weed

SCIENTIFIC NAME: Chimaphila maculata

LOCAL NAME: Rat's Vein (Spotted Pipsissewa)

LEE'S CLASSIFICATION: MT MR A

USE(S): Heart trouble, poor appetite

ACTIVE INGREDIENTS:
Chimaphilin and arbutin. (*Hagers:* 853)

Arbutin. (*FNF:* 146)

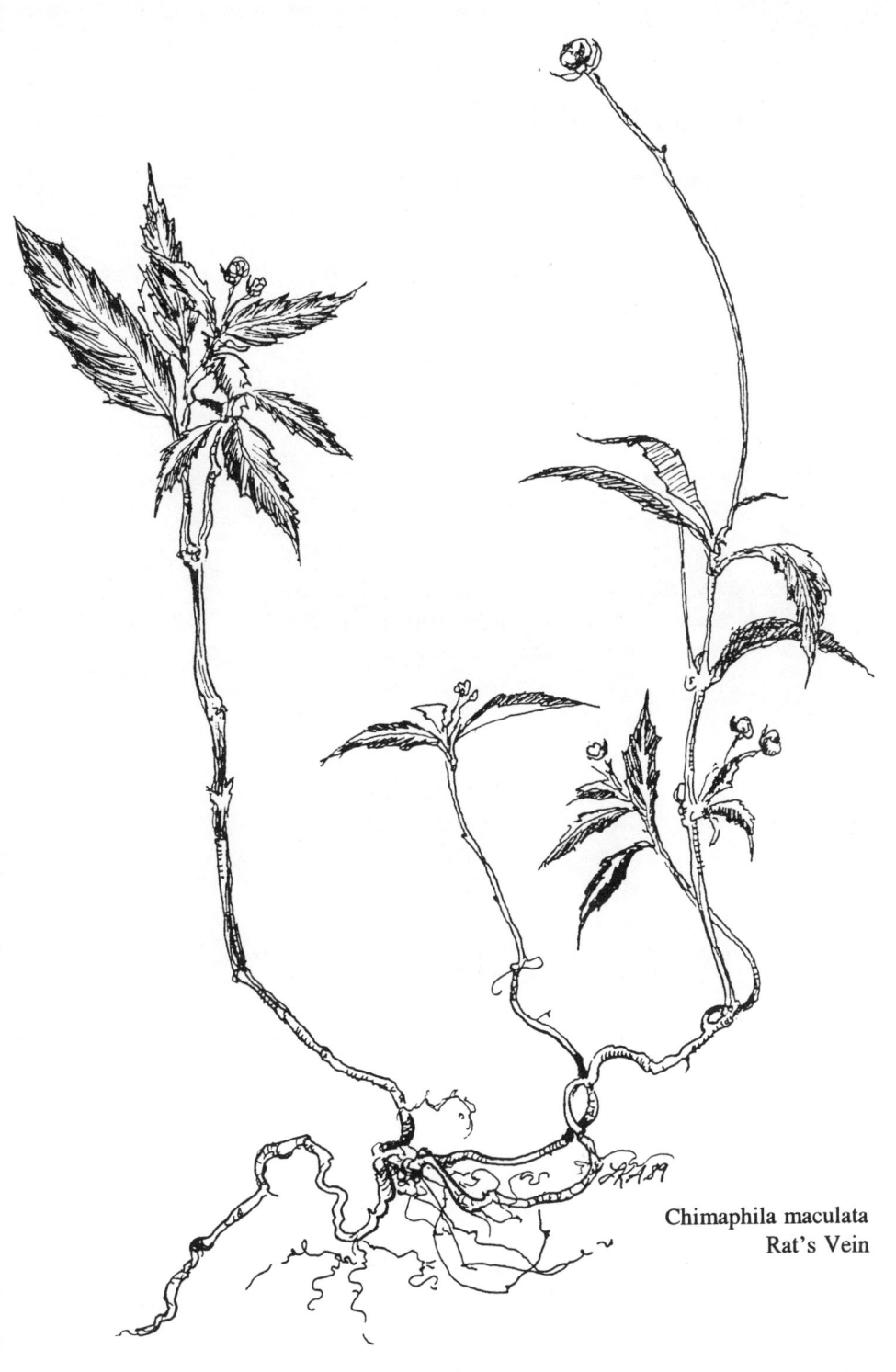

Chimaphila maculata
Rat's Vein

SCIENTIFIC NAME: Cimicifuga racemosa

LOCAL NAME: Black Cohosh

LEE'S CLASSIFICATION: ST VSR VA

USE(S): Bronchitis, arthritis, rheumatism, fever, diabetes, prostate gland, heart trouble, stomach trouble, blood purifier, diarrhea, swelling, aphrodisiac, menstrual cramps, loss of appetite

ACTIVE INGREDIENTS:
Dry seeds: alkaloid N-methylcytisine and other unnamed alkaloids; Root: amorphous resinous substance called cimicifugin (macrotin) and racemosin (bitter principle). Two triterpene glycosides, actein, and cimigoside. Two resins and an astrigent principle. Acetic, butyric, formic, oleic, tannic, gallic, salicylic, palmitic, and isoferulic acids. (Duke: 121)

Acetic acid, actein, butyric acid, cimicifugin, cimigenol- xyloside, 27-desoxyacetylacteol, fat, formic acid, gallic acid, isoferulic acid, N-methylcytisine, oleic acid, palmitic acid, protein, resin, racemosin, salicylic acid, tannic acid, tannin. (*FNF:* 151-52)

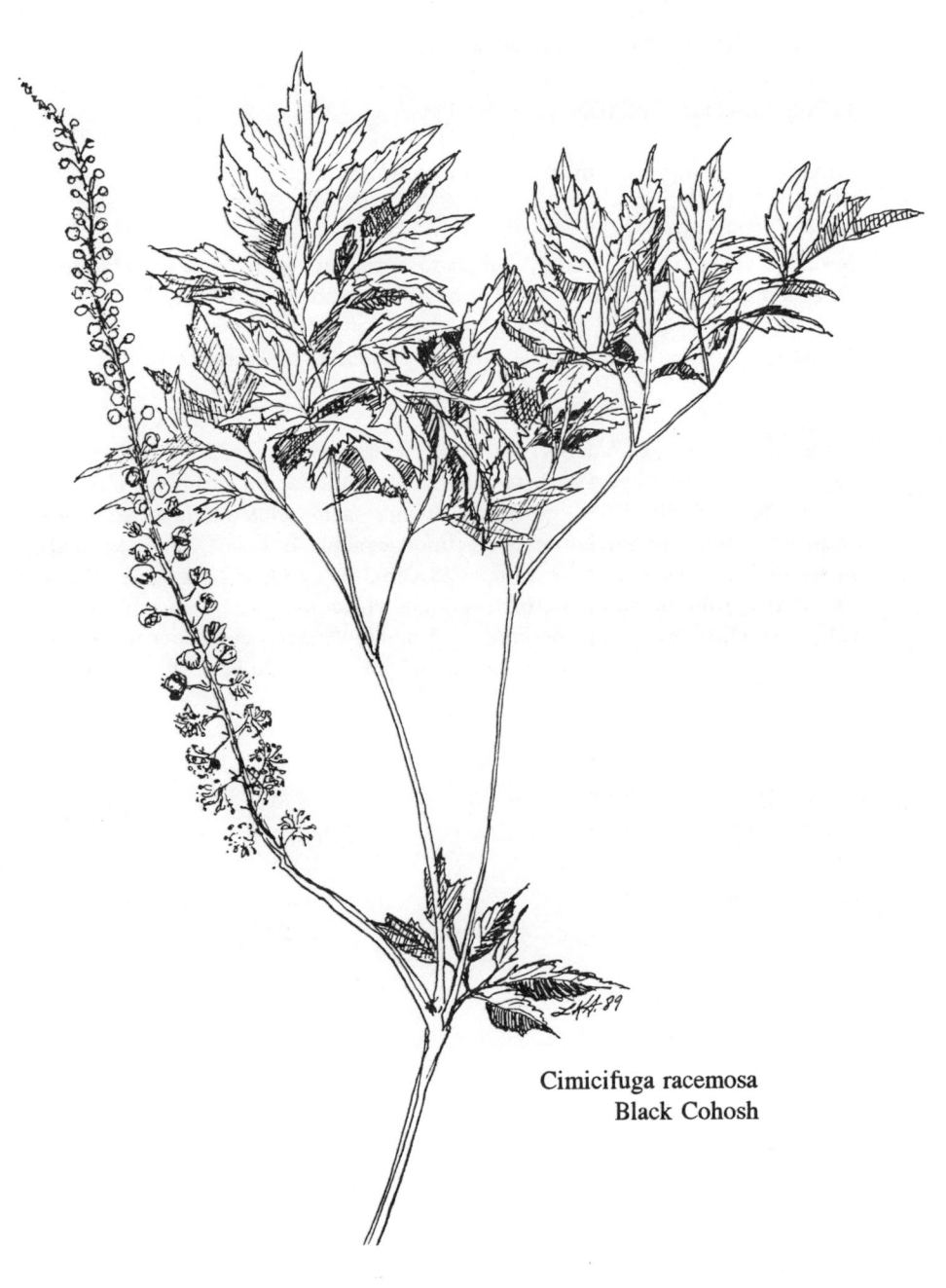

Cimicifuga racemosa
Black Cohosh

SCIENTIFIC NAME: Citrullus lanatus

LOCAL NAME: Watermelon Seeds

LEE'S CLASSIFICATION: MT SR VA

USE(S): Urinary tract infection, poor blood circulation

ACTIVE INGREDIENTS:
Seeds: phyto sterolin (ipurano), two phytosterols, two hydrocarbons, a saponin, an alkaloid, a polysaccharide or glycoside, and tannin. (*FNF:* 160-61)

Glutelin, globulin, water soluble protein, proteosis, peptones. (*Wealth of Ind:* 187)

Alpha-amino-beta-(1-imidazoyl)-propionic acid, arginine, calcium, capric acid, caprylic acid, carbohydrate, beta-carotene, citrullic acid, citrulline, citrullol, cucur-bitacin-E, fat, fiber, globulin, glutamic acid, glutelin, hentriacontane, iron, L-(+)-isoleucine, lauric acid, linoleic acid, lycopene, myristic acid, neolycopene, neurosporin, niacin, CIS,CIS-3,6-nonadien-1-OL, oleic acid, oxysilvine, palmitic acid, pectin, L-(-)-phenylalanine, phosphorus, physetolic acid, poly-CIS-lycopene, potassium, pro-beta-carotene, proneurosporin, protein, L-beta-(pyrazol- 1-YL)-alanine, riboflavin, sodium, stearic acid, thiamin, L-(-)-threonine, L-(-)-tyrosine, urease, (+)-valine, water. (*FNF:* 160-61)

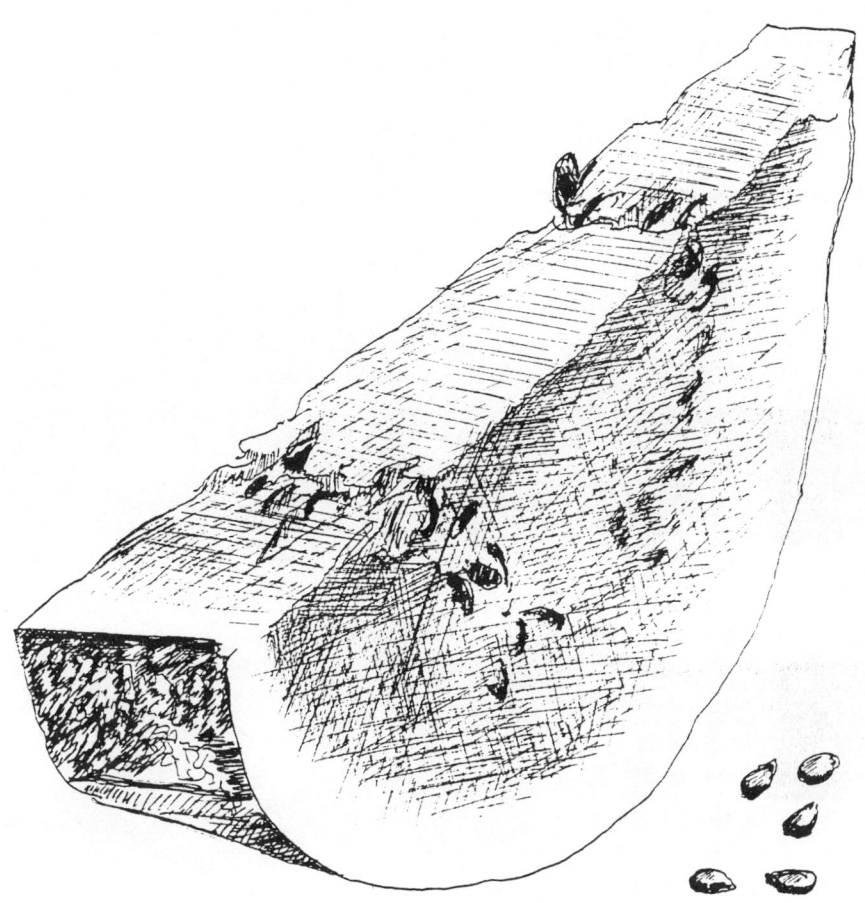

Citrullus lanatus
Watermelon

SCIENTIFIC NAME: Cynoglossum virginianum

LOCAL NAME: Wild Comfrey

LEE'S CLASSIFICATION: ST MR A

USE(S):   Ulcers, menstrual cramps, colds, wounds, swelling, diarrhea, gout

ACTIVE INGREDIENTS:
Alkaloid: cynoglossine. (Felter and Lloyd: 642)

Some alkaloids in this family are carcinogenic. (Duke: personal communication)

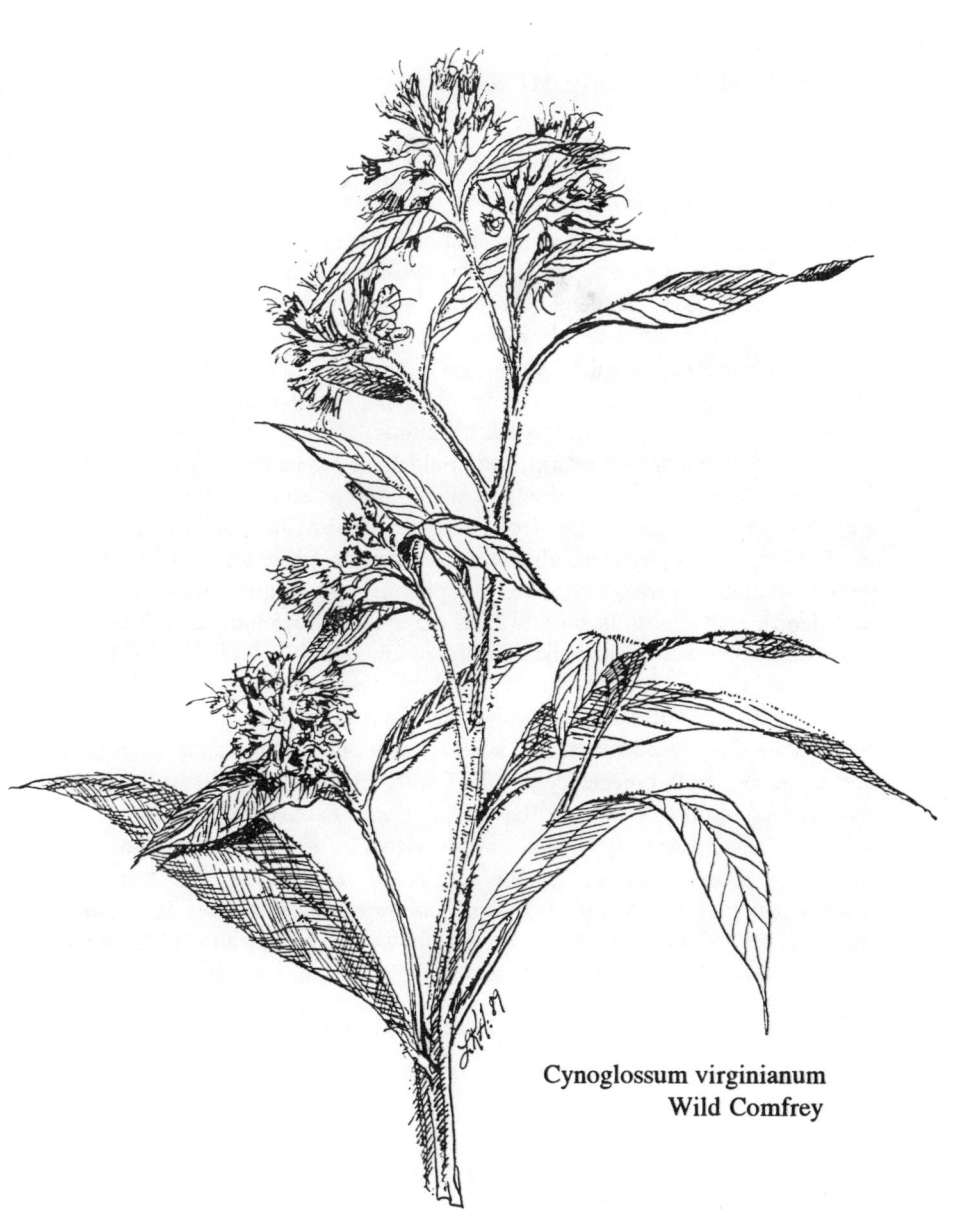

Cynoglossum virginianum
Wild Comfrey

SCIENTIFIC NAME: Daucus carota

LOCAL NAME: Queen Anne's Lace (carrot)

LEE'S CLASSIFICATION: MT SR VA

USE(S): Menstrual cramps, gas

ACTIVE INGREDIENTS:
Acetone, acetylcholine, acorenone, aluminum, apigenin-4'-0-beta-D-glycoside, apigenin-7-0-beta-d-galactopyranosyl-(1,4)-0-beta-D-mann, arsenic, asarone, ascorbic acid, ash, azulene, barium, bergamotene, cis-beta-bergamotene, bergapten, beta-bisabolene, bornyl-acetate, boron, butyric acid, cadmium, calcium, camphene, camphor, carbohydrates, delta-3-carene, carotatoxin, beta-carotene, carotol, carvone, caryophyllene, alpha-caryophyllene, beta-caryophyllene, caryophyllene-oxide, chromium, citral, citric acid, citronellyl-acetate, cobalt, copper, coumarin, cumin-aldehyde, alpha-curcumene, P-cymene, P-cymol, daucene, daucic acid, daucol, daucosterol, gamma-decalactose, gamma-decanolactone, diosgenin, dipentene, beta-elemene, epoxydihydrocaryophyllene, ethanol, farnesene, fat, fiber, formic acid, geraniol, geranyl-acetate, geranyl-formate, D-glucose, glutamine, alpha-gurjunene, heraclenin, HCN, iron, isobutyric acid, isopimpinellin, kaempferol-3-0-beta-D-glucoside, alpha-ketogluitaric acid, lead, lecithin, lecithinase, limonene, linalool, linoleic acid, lithium, lycopene, magnesium, malic acid, maltose, manganese, mercury, molybdenum, myrcene, myristicin, niacin, nickle, 2-octanone, osthole, oxalic acid, oxypeucedanin, palmitic acid, pectin, phosphorus, phytin, phytoene, alpha-pinene, beta-pinene, pipecolic acid, potassium, protein, psoralen, pyrrolidine, quinic acid, riboflavin, sabinene, saccharose, selenium, beta-selinene, beta-sitosterol, beta-sitosterol-gylcoside, sodium, strontium, sulfur, terpinen, alpha-terpinene, gamma-terpinene, alpha-terpineol, terpinolene, thiamin, tin, titanium, tocopherol, trans-beta-bergaptene, trans-1,10-heptadeca-diene-5,7-diyn-3-OL,trans-2,(7)-2,6-fimethylocta-4,6-diene,umbelliferone,vitamin D, vitamin E, water, xanthotoxin, zinc, zirconium, zosimin. (*FNF:* 214-16)

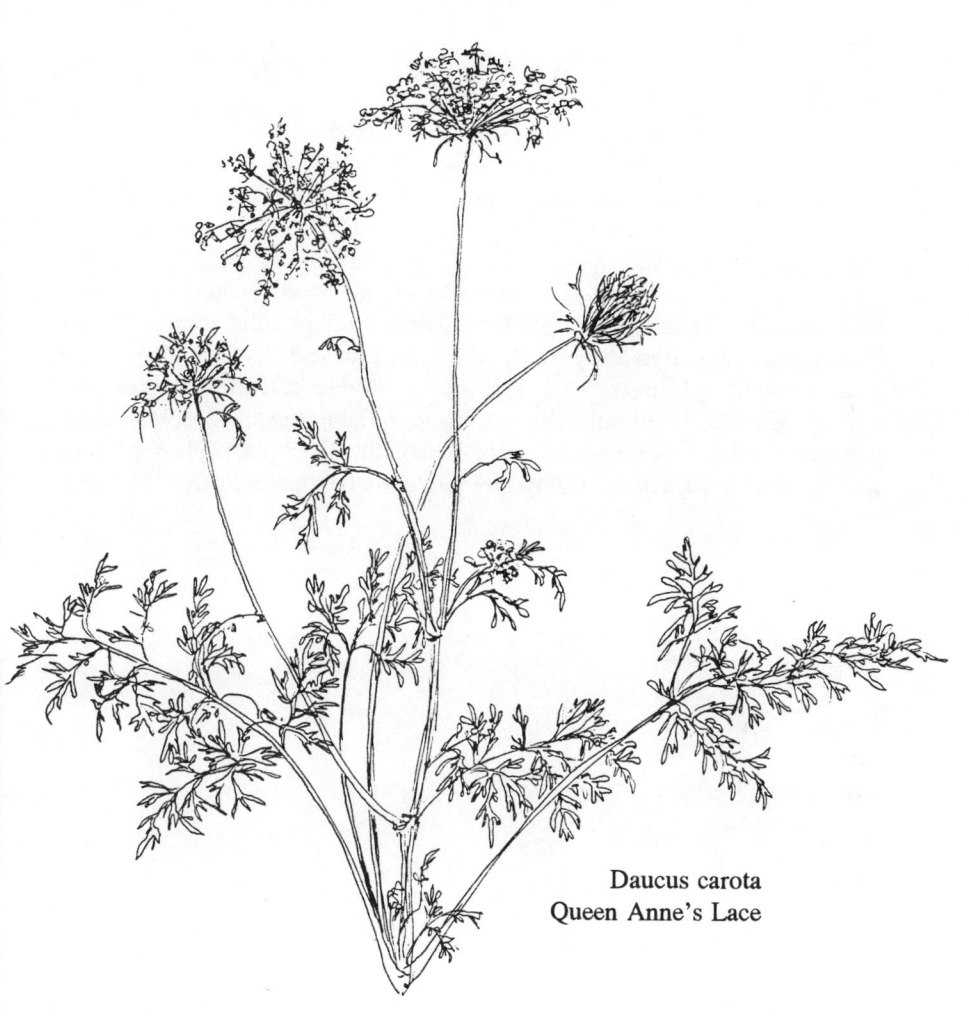
Daucus carota
Queen Anne's Lace

SCIENTIFIC NAME: Datura stramonium

LOCAL NAME: Jimsonweed

LEE'S CLASSIFICATION: ___ VSR VA Powerful

USE(S): Sores

ACTIVE INGREDIENTS:
Hyposcyamine, scopalamine, atropine. (Duke: 162)

Acetic acid, acetone, aconitic acid, aesculetin, alkaloids, ascorbic acid, atropamine, atropine, atropinesterase, utanol, caffeic acid, chlorogenic acid, citric acid, cuscohygrine, datugen, datugenin, ditigloyl-D-dehydroxy-tropane, 3-alpha,6-beta-ditigloyloxytropane, EO, ethanol, fat, ferulic acid, formaldehyde, formic acid, fumaric acid, galactose, glucose, glycolic acid, hyoscine, hyoscyamine, isobutyraldehyde, alpha-ketoglutaric acid, lactic acid, lignoceric acid, linoleic acid, meteloidin, malic acid, methanol, neochlorogenic acid, nicotine, oleic acid, palmitic acid, potassium-nitrate, propionaldehyde, protein, putrescine, rutin, scopin, scopalamine, scopoletin, sitosterol, sophorose, stearic acid, succinic acid, tannin, tigloylmeteloidin, umbelliferone. (*FNF:* 213-14)

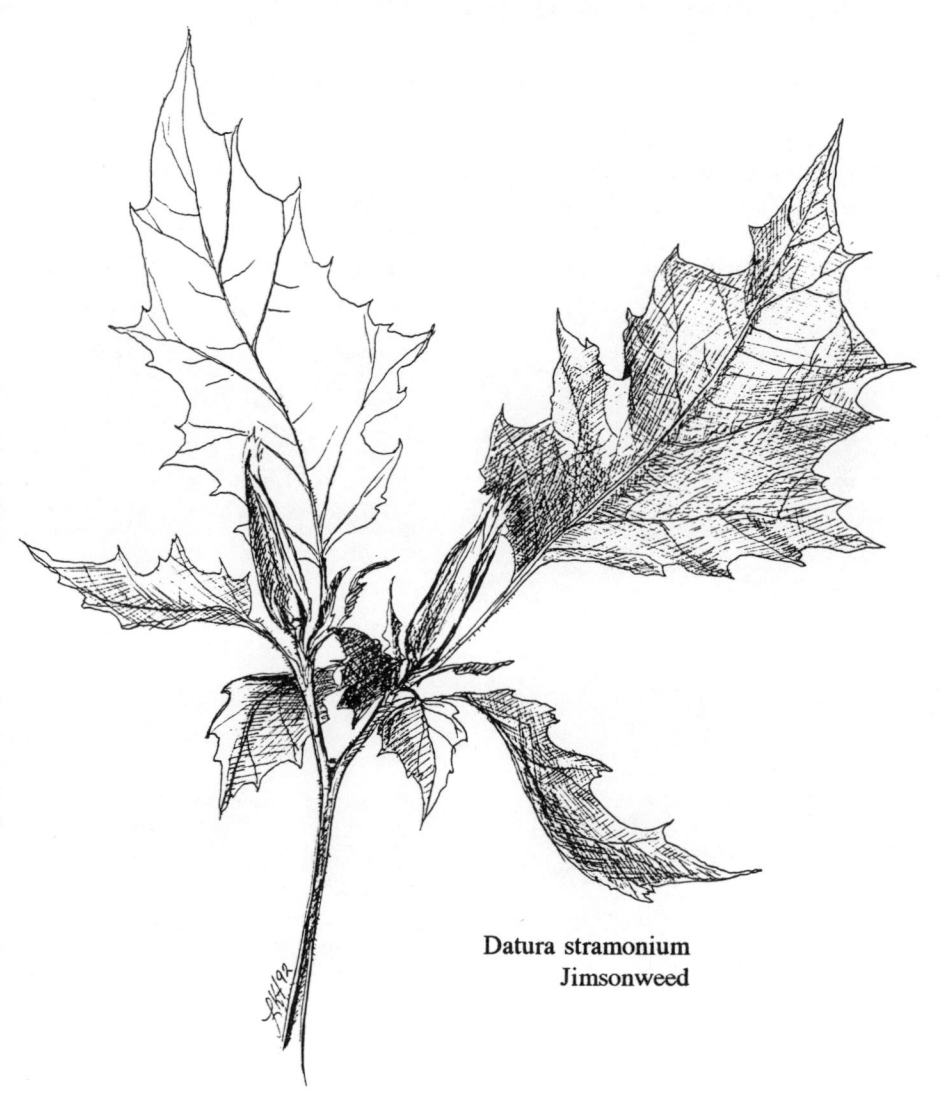

Datura stramonium
Jimsonweed

SCIENTIFIC NAME: Eupatorium perfoliatum

LOCAL NAME: Boneset

LEE'S CLASSIFICATION: ST SR A

USE(S): Colds, flu, pneumonia, fluid in the lungs, fevers, coughs

ACTIVE INGREDIENTS:
Eupatorin, tannic acid, gallic acid, a bitter glucoside, resin, gum, a volatile oil. Various flavonoids, sterols, and triterpenes. (Duke: 188)

Eupatorin, gallic-acid, gum, 4-0-methylglucuronoxylan, resin, tannic-acid. (*FNF:* 231)

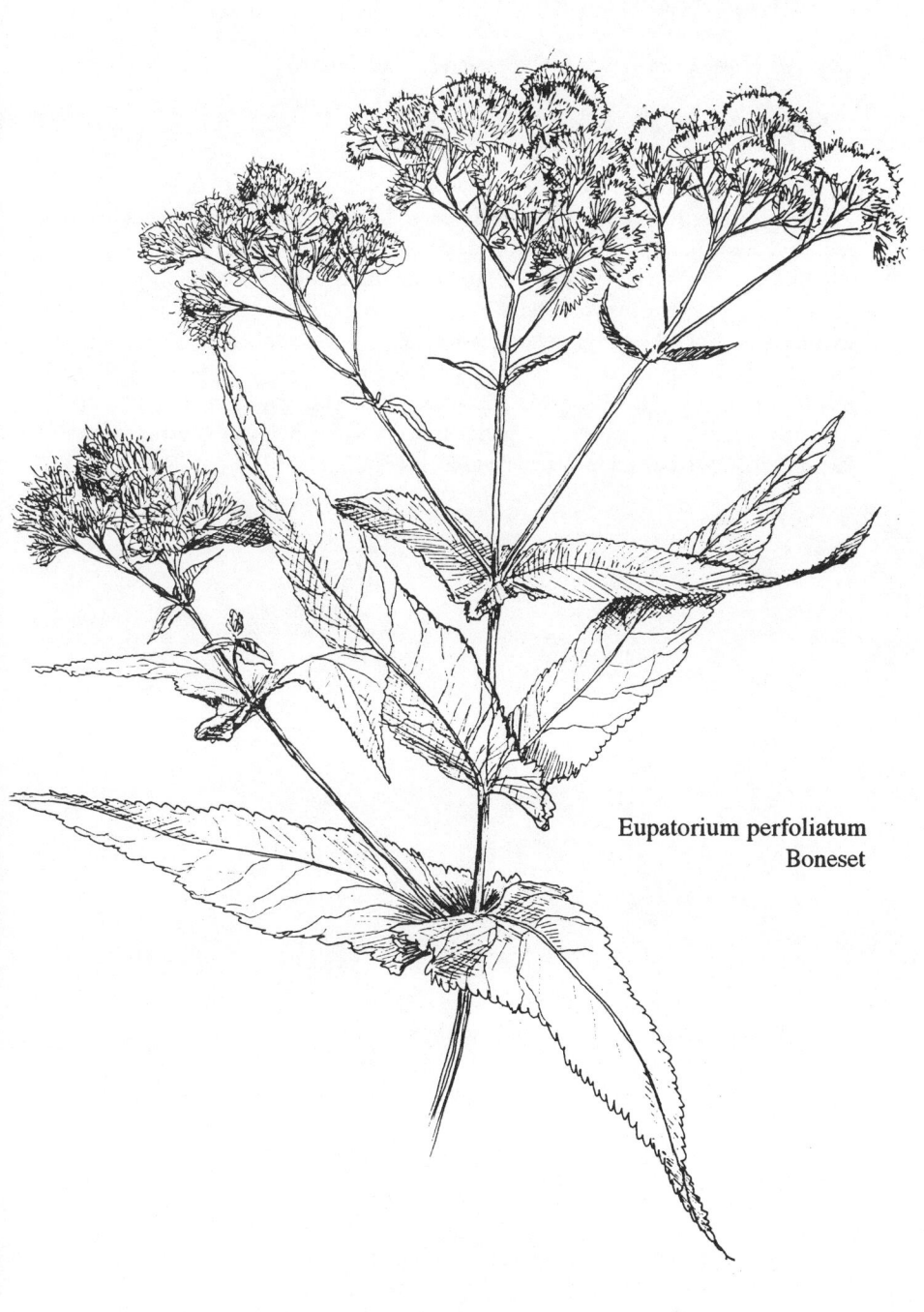

Eupatorium perfoliatum
Boneset

SCIENTIFIC NAME: Euphorbia hirta

LOCAL NAME: Milkweed (Queensland asthma herb)

USE(S): Sores, cuts, warts

ACTIVE INGREDIENTS:
20-0-acetylreseniferenol-9,13,14-orthophenylacetate,alpha-amyrin,beta-amyrin, ascorbic acid, betulin, campesterol, camphol, caoutchouc, chlorophenolic acid, cholesterol, choline, P-coumaric acid, cyanidin-3,5-diglucoside, cycloartenol, 12-deoxy-4-beta-hydroxyphorbol-13-dodecanoate-20-acetate, 12-deoxy-4-beta-hydroxyphorbol-13-phenylacetate-20-acetate, 12-deoxyphorbol-13-phenyl-acetate-16-0-alpha-methyletc, 3,4 dioxyphenylalanine, ellagic acid, euphorbol-hexocosonate, fat, ferulic acid, friedelan, friedelin, gallic acid, gum, HCN, hentriacontane, L-hexacosanol, ingenol-triacetate, inositol, jambulol, kaempferol, kaempferol-3-glucuronide, leucocyanidol. (*FNF:* 231-32)

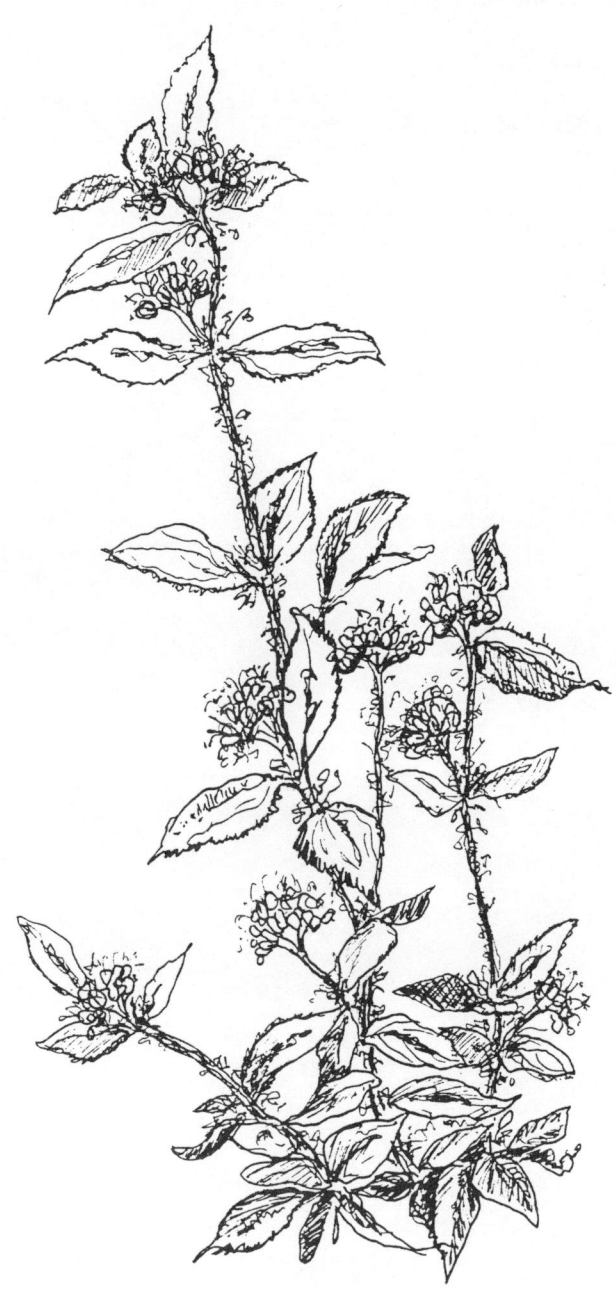

Euphorbia hirta
Milkweed

SCIENTIFIC NAME: Gaylussacia spp.

LOCAL NAME: Huckleberry

LEE'S CLASSIFICATION: MT MR A

USE(S): Diabetes

ACTIVE INGREDIENTS:
No references found for this herb.

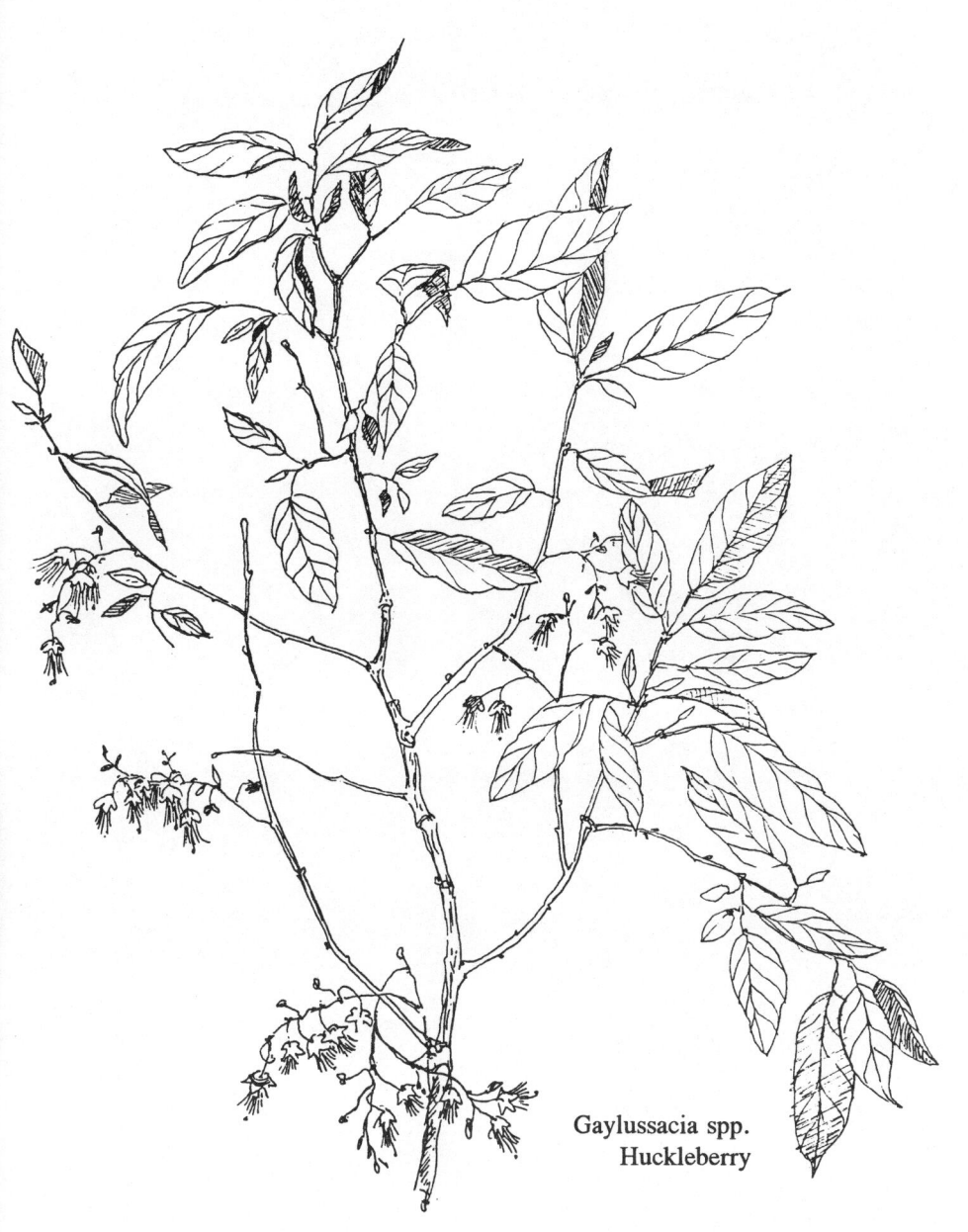
Gaylussacia spp.
Huckleberry

SCIENTIFIC NAME: Gnaphalium obtusifolium

LOCAL NAME: Rabbit Tobacco

LEE'S CLASSIFICATION: VST SR VA

USE(S): Asthma, headaches, colds, mucus buildup

ACTIVE INGREDIENTS:
Gnaphaliin, 5,7,-dihydroxy-3,8-dimethoxyflavon, 3-mono-methylather, obtusifolin,3,5,7-trihydroxy-6,8-dimethoxy-flavon. (*Hagers:* 1177)

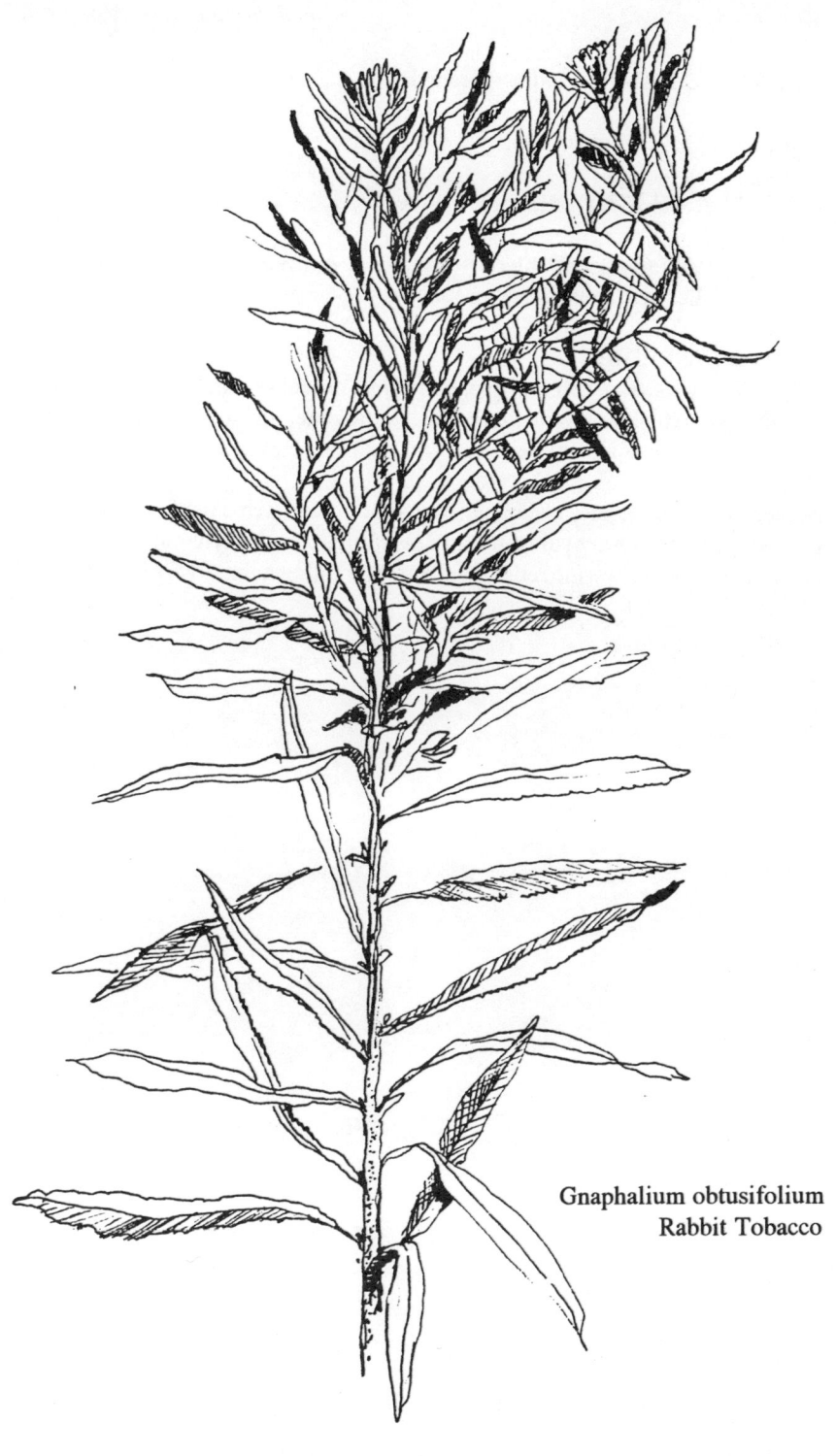

Gnaphalium obtusifolium
Rabbit Tobacco

SCIENTIFIC NAME: Hydrastis canadensis

LOCAL NAME: Golden Seal

LEE'S CLASSIFICATION: MT MR A

USE(S): Bad (unclean) blood, arthritis, stomach trouble, constipation, allergies, gout, sinus problems

ACTIVE INGREDIENTS:
Alkaloids: hydrastine, berberastine, berberine, canadine, candaline, hydrastinine, 5-hydroxytetrahydrobeberine, meconine, reticuline, and xanthopucine; Volatile oils: chlorogenic acid, phytosterins, and resins. (Duke: 239)

Berberastine, berberine, canadine, candaline, chlorogenic acid, D-fructose, D-galactose, D-glucose, hydrastine, hydrastinine, 5-hydroxytetrahydroberberine, inositol, meconine, resin, reticuline, starch, xanthopucine. (*FNF:* 287)

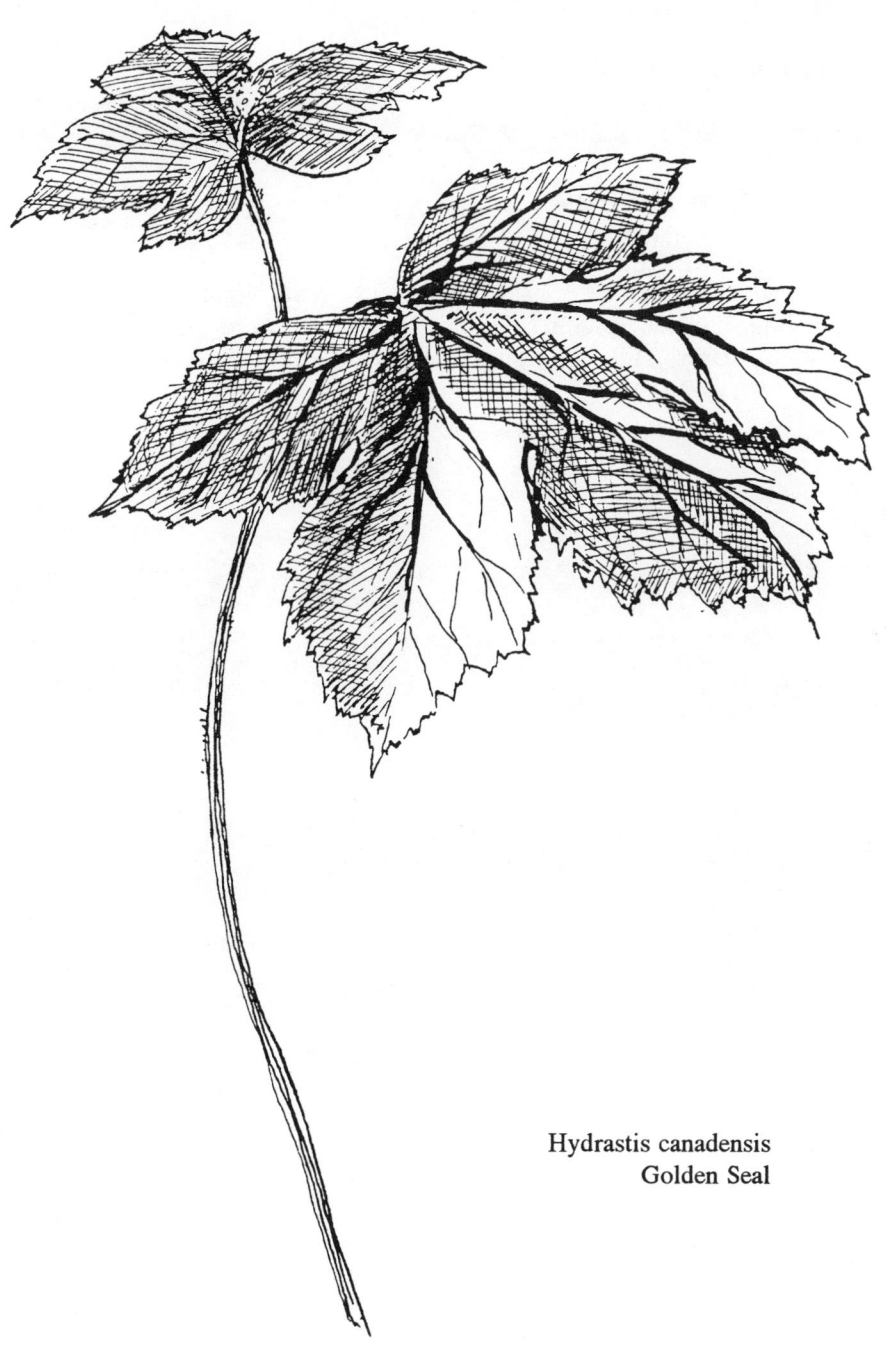

Hydrastis canadensis
Golden Seal

SCIENTIFIC NAME: Lactuca spp.

LOCAL NAME: Milkweed (Wild Lettuce)

LEE'S CLASSIFICATION: ___ VSR VA

USE(S): Sores, cuts, warts

ACTIVE INGREDIENTS:
Some species of lactuca contain choline, citric acid, ergosterol, folic acid, hyoscyamine, malic acid, oxalic acid, pectin, latucerin (alpha- and beta-lactucerol); Dried Milk: lactucopicrin, lactucin, lactucic acid, and lactuceral. (Duke: 264; *FNF:* 310)

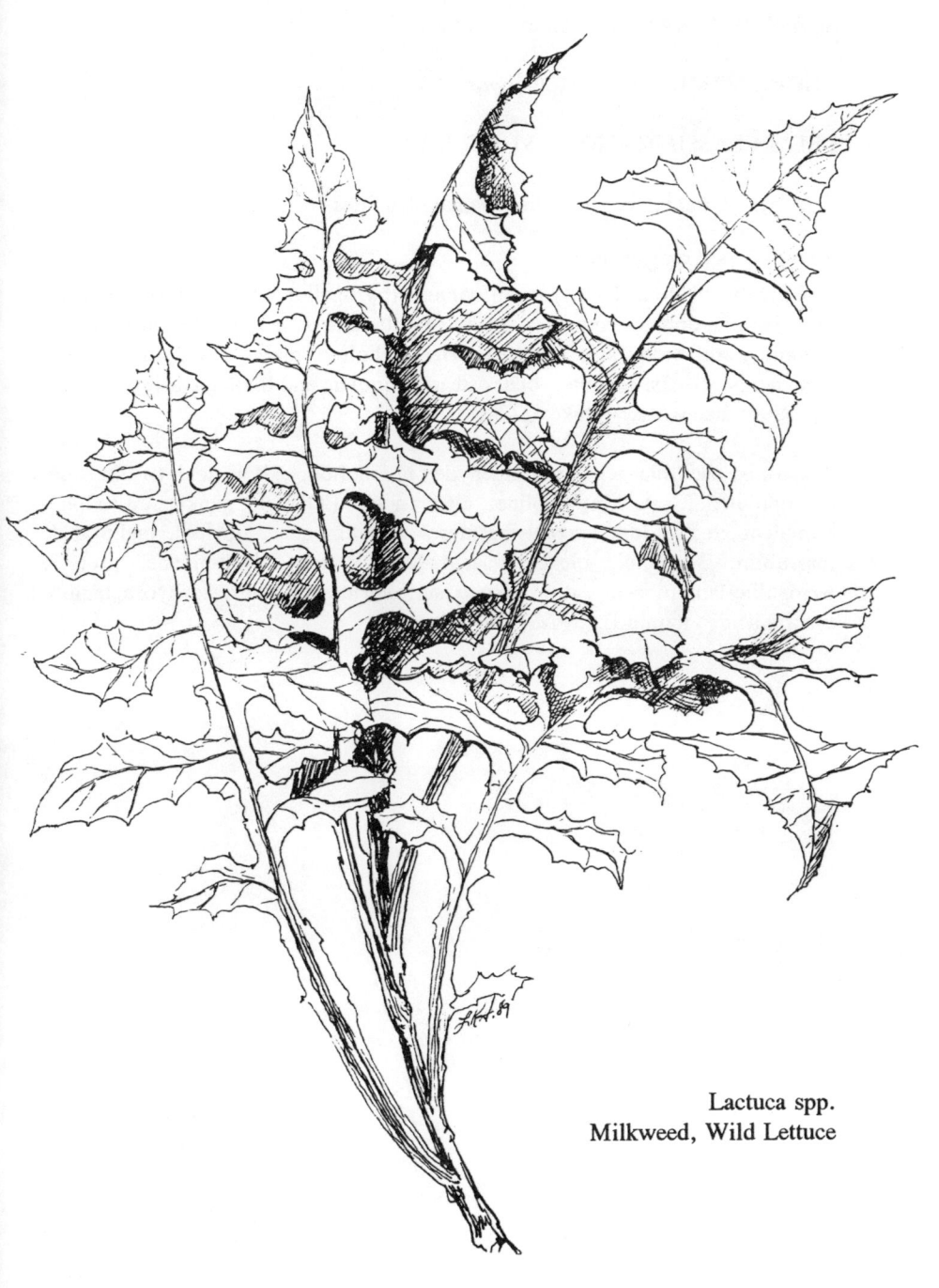

Lactuca spp.
Milkweed, Wild Lettuce

SCIENTIFIC NAME: Leonurus cardiaca

LOCAL NAME: Balm (Motherwort)

LEE'S CLASSIFICATION: ST MR VA

USE(S): Urinary tract infection, female troubles

ACTIVE INGREDIENTS:
Dry plants: alkaloids (stachydrine), tannins (pyrogallol and catechins), essential oils, carbohydrates, saponins, traces of vitamins A and C, leonurin resins, saponins, and waxes also reported. Herb: choline, malic, citric, ursolic, and oleic acids; Seeds: palmitic, oleic, stearic, linoleic and linolenic acids, vitamin E; Root: stachyose. (Duke: 277-28)

Alkaloids, ascorbic acid, benzaldehyde, bufenolide, caffeic-acid-4-rutinoside, caryophyllene, catechin, choline, citric acid, EO, fat, genkwanin, alpha-humulene, leonur-idine, leonurine uterotonic, limonene, linalool, malic acid, marrubiin, 3-octanol, oleanolic acid, alpha-pinene, beta-pinene, protein, pyrogallic-tannin, resin, rutin, saponin, stachydrine oxytocic?, stachyose, tannin, ursolic acid, vitamin E. (*FNF:* 319-20)

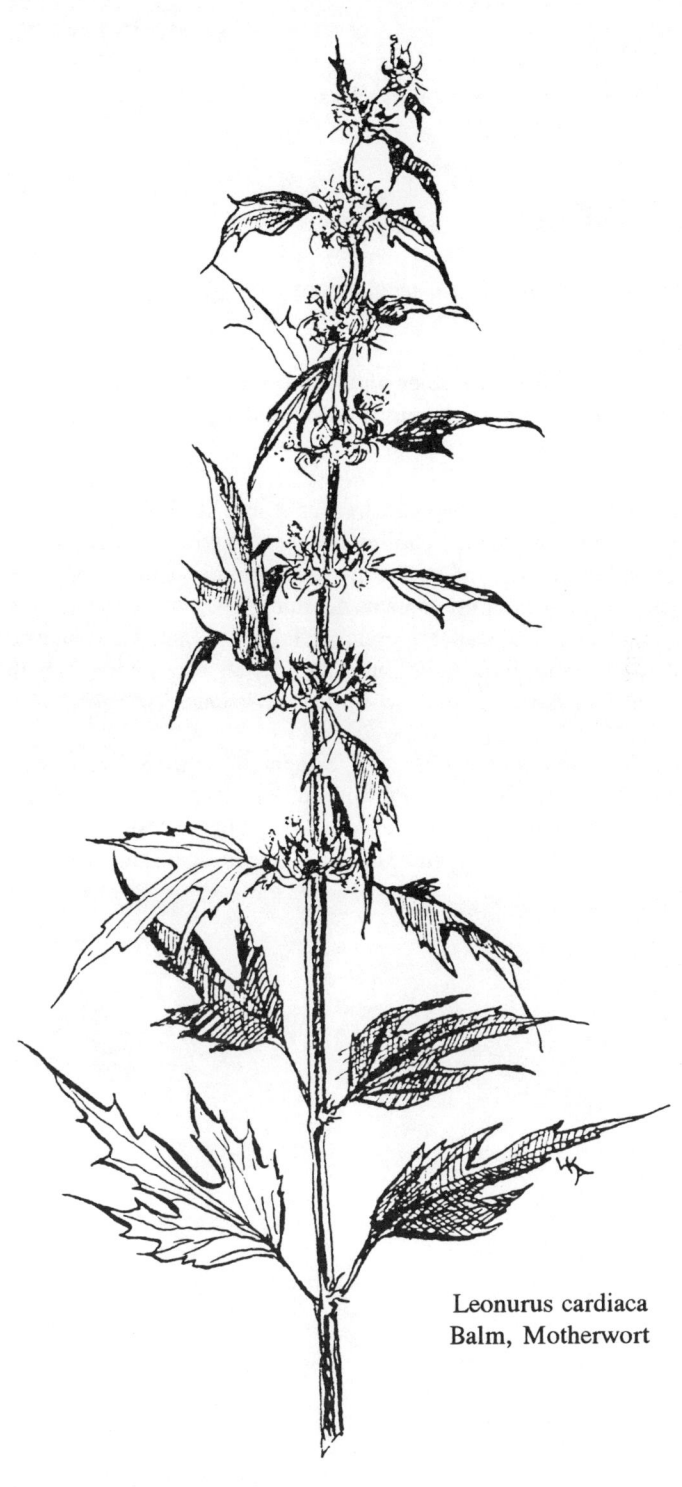

Leonurus cardiaca
Balm, Motherwort

SCIENTIFIC NAME: Marrubium vulgare (cultivated)

LOCAL NAME: Horehound

LEE'S CLASSIFICATION: ST SR A

USE(S): Chest colds, asthma, chicken pox

ACTIVE INGREDIENTS:
Plant contains marrubiin together with other bitter principles and volatile oil, ursolic acid, a resin, a wax, tannin, mucilage, a saponin, and choline. (*Wealth of Ind.*: 305)

Diterpine, marrubiin, diterpenoidmarrubenol and its hemiacetal; tannic acid, beta-sitosterol, beta-glucoside, choline, and beonienkraut; marrubiin forms as an artifact out of premarrubiin; stachydrine, flavonoids, anthocyane, Vitamin C, caffeic acid. An essential oil contains sesquiterpene; tannin, gallic, and ursolic acid, mucila-ginous substances, and pectin, resin and wax substance with unsaturated fat sterol; diterpenoid, marrubiol, N-alkanes 2-bzw, 3-methylakane, 2(w-1)-di-methyalkane,3,9, or 3,(w-9)-dimethylalkane. (*Hagers:* 704)

Ascorbic acid, betonicine, caffeic acid, camphene, choline, P-cymene, EO, fat, gallic acid, limonene, marrubenol, marrubiin, marrubiol, mucilage, pectin, peregrinol, alpha-pinene, protein, resin, sabinene, beta-sitosterol, beta-sitosterol-beta-glucoside, tannic acid, tannin, turicine, ursolic acid, vulgarol, wax. (*FNF:* Vol.2: 9)

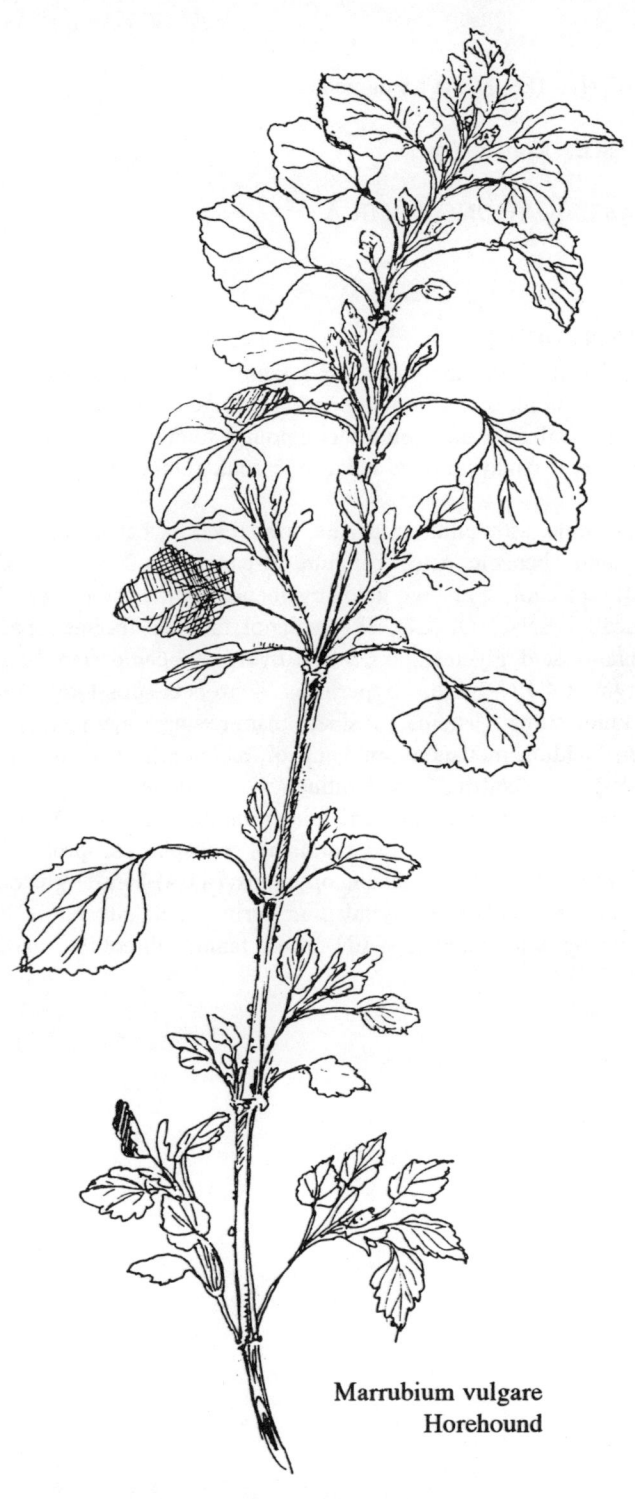

Marrubium vulgare
Horehound

SCIENTIFIC NAME: Melia azedarach

LOCAL NAME: Chinaberry

LEE'S CLASSIFICATION: ST MR A

USE(S): Worms

ACTIVE INGREDIENTS:
Leaves: paraisine; Bark: margosine and tannin; Fruit: azadirine and resin; glycerides of palmitic, oleic, linoleic, and stearic acids; azadirachtin. Vanillic acid, an ascaricidal and anthelmintic compound found in the cortex with dicatechol; Pericarp: bakayanin and bakayanic acid. (Duke: 304)

Alkaloids, arginine, astragalin, azadarine, azadarachtin, bakalactone, bakayanic acid, bakayanin, benzoic acid, calcium, 4-campesten-3-one, carbohydrate, catechin, DL-catechol, cinnamic acid, cycloeucalenol, cystine, 21,23, 24,25-diepoxi-tirucall-7-EN-21-OL, EO, EPI-melianol, fat fiber, fraxinellone, gedunin, glucose, glutamic acid, glycine, gum, 3-beta-hydroxy-5-campesten-7-one, 6-beta-hydroxy-stigmast-4-EN-3-one, hyperin, 7-keto-beta-sitos-terol, kulactone, kulinone, kulolactone, leucine, lysine, mangrovine, margosine, melanol, meldenin, meliandiol, melianone, meliantriol, meliatoxin-A-1, meliatoxin-A-2, meliatoxin-B-1, melicitrin, methionine, 24-methylenecyclo-artanol, 24-methylenecycloartenone, nimbin, nimbinin, nimbiol, nimbolin-A, nimbolin-B, ochcinal, ohchinin, palmitic acid, paraisine, phosphorus, proline, protein, quercitrin, resin, 7-0-alpha-L-rhamnopyranosyl-(1-4)-beta-D-glucopyranosil, rutin, saponin, sedanolactone, sendanin, serine, beta-sitosterol-3-0-beta-D-glucoside, stearic acid, stigmast-4-EN-3-one, tannin, threonine, vanillic acid, vanillin. (*FNF:* 13-15)

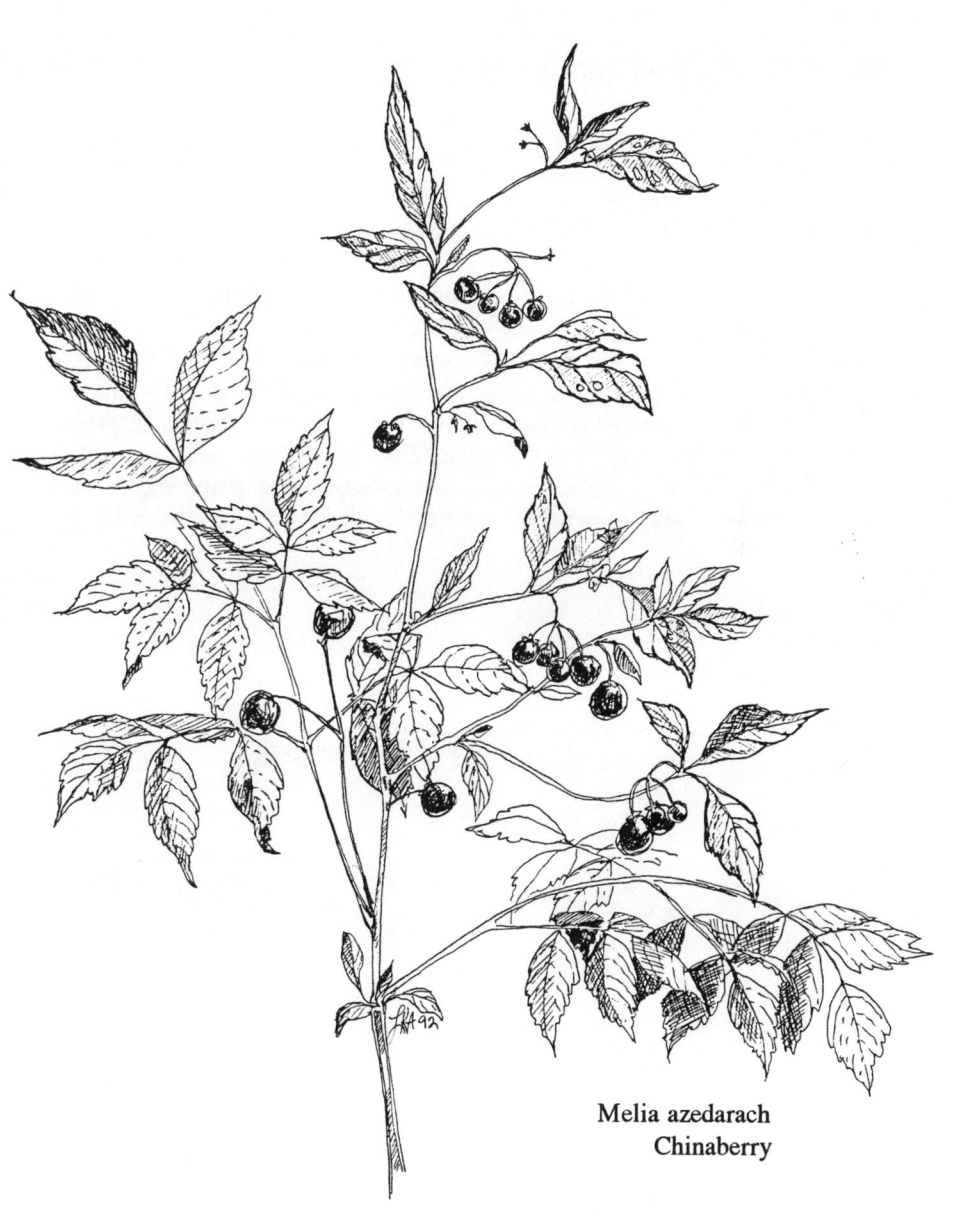

Melia azedarach
Chinaberry

SCIENTIFIC NAME: Melissa officinalis

LOCAL NAME: Lemon Mint (Balm)

LEE'S CLASSIFICATION: MT SR VA

USE(S): Stomach problems, insomnia

ACTIVE INGREDIENTS:
Tannin, gum, stearopten. (Felter and Lloyd: 1252-53)

Beta-bourbonene, delta-cadinene, gamma-cadinene, 10-alpha-cadinol, caffeic acid, caryophyllene, caryophyllene-oxide, catechins, chlorogenic acid, citral-A, citral-B, citro-nellal, (+)-citronellal, copaene, alpha-cubebene, EO, eugenol-acetate, fat, geranial, geraniol, geranyl-acetate, germacrene-D, CIS-3-hexenol, alpha-humulene, isogeranial, linalool, luteolin-7-glucoside, methyl-heptenone, neral, nerol, CIS-ocimene, trans-ocimene, 3-octanol, 3-octanone, 1-octen-3-OL, octyl-benzoate, oleanolic-acid, protein, protocatechuic acid, rhamnazin, rosmaric acid, rosmarinic acid, stachyose, succinic acid, thymol, ursolic acid, wax. (*FNF:* 15-16)

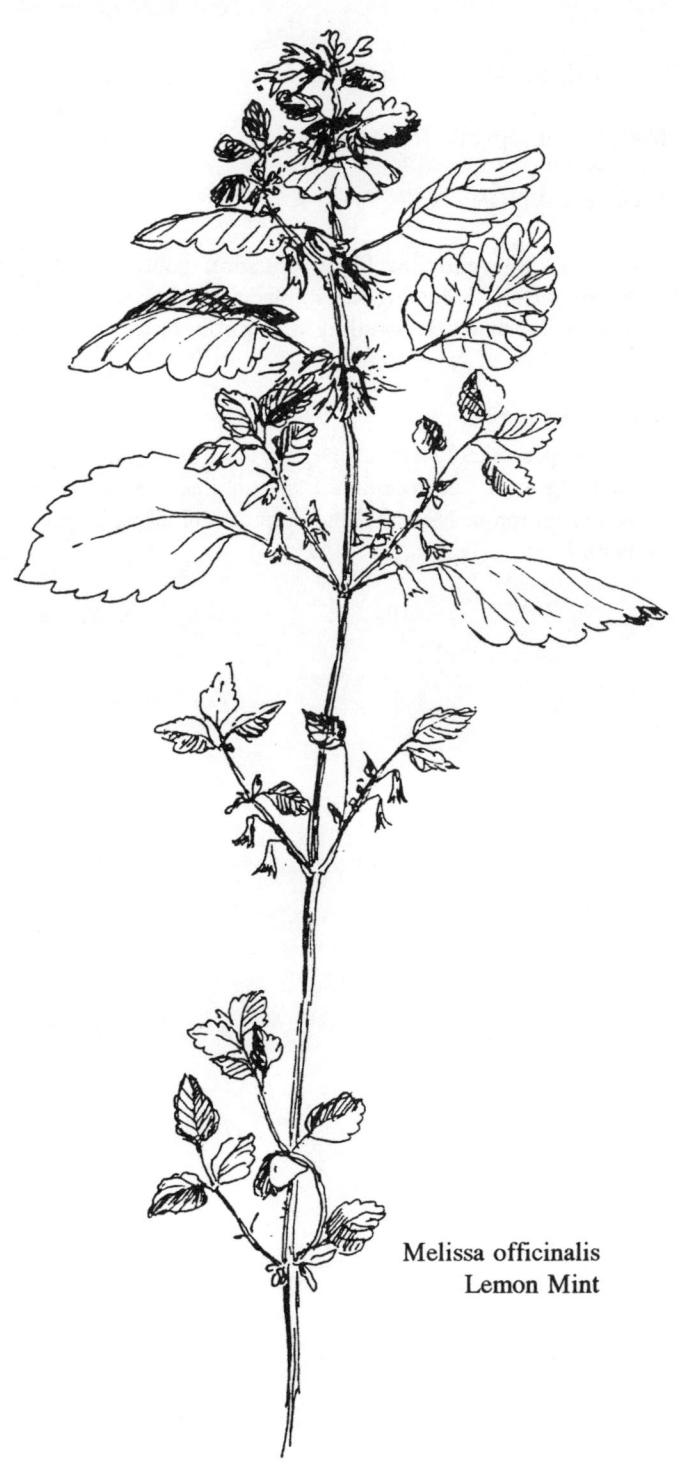

Melissa officinalis
Lemon Mint

SCIENTIFIC NAME: Menispermum canadense

LOCAL NAME: Sarsaparilla (Moonseed)

LEE'S CLASSIFICATION: VST VSR VA

USE(S): Diabetes, high and low blood pressure, gout, arthritis, earaches, prostate gland, kidney problems, bladder and urinary tract problems, styes, boils, diarrhea, swelling, dandruff, sore or weak eyes, heart murmur, loss of appetite

ACTIVE INGREDIENTS:
Alkaloid dauricine, presumably tetrandrine, and viburmitol; Above ground parts: acutumine, the rhizome acutomidine, daurinoline, N-desmethyldauricin, magnoflorine, and aporphine N-methyllind-carpinmethiodide, the protoverberine dehydrocheilanthifoline. (Duke: 224; *FNF:* 16)

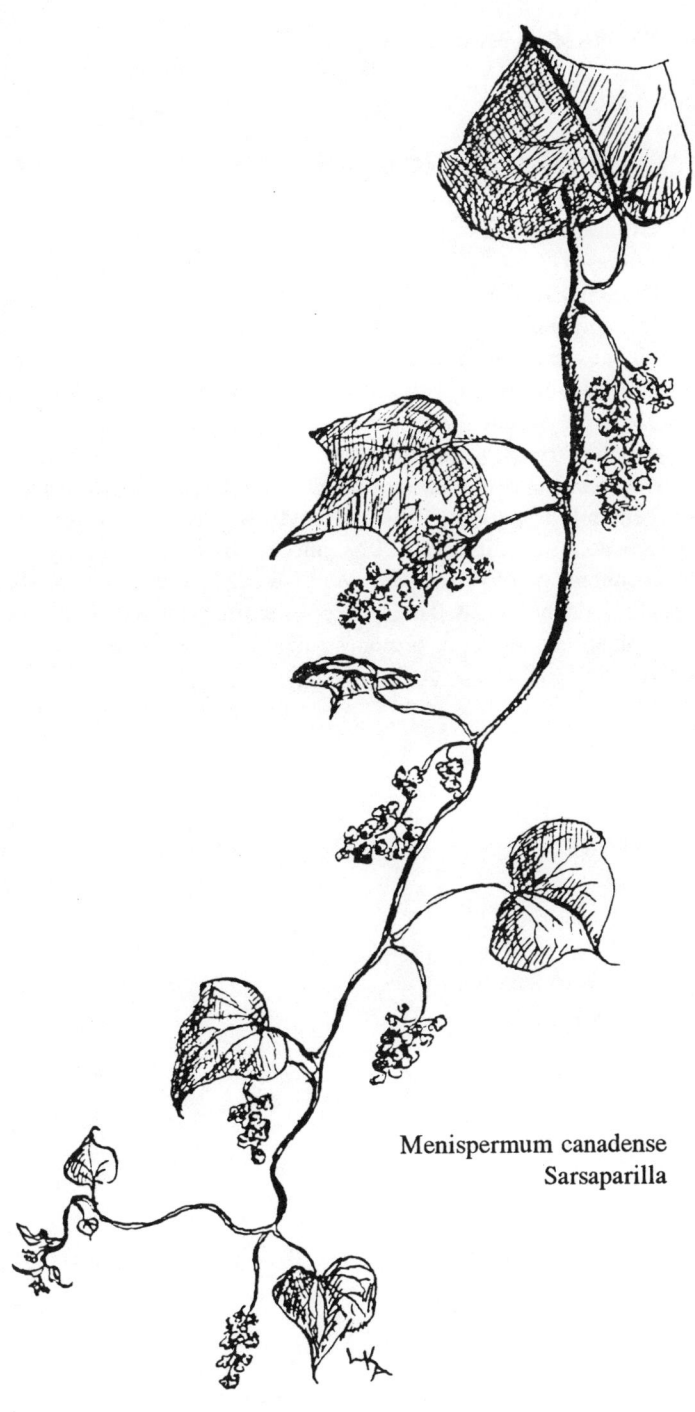

Menispermum canadense
Sarsaparilla

SCIENTIFIC NAME: Mentha spp.

LOCAL NAME: Mint

LEE'S CLASSIFICATION: MT SR A

USE(S): Stomach troubles

ACTIVE INGREDIENTS:
Acetic acid, apigenin, ash, beta-bourbonene, butyric acid, delta-cadinene, gamma-cadinene, cadinol, calcium, camphene, caproic acid, caprylic acid, carbohydrate, beta-carotene, carvacrol, CIS-carveol, trans-carveol, carvone-acetate, CIS-carvyl-acetate, trans-carvyl-acetate, caryophyllene, 1,8,-cineole, copper, dihydrocarveol, dihydrocarvone, dihydrocarvyl-acetate, diosmin, diosmetin-7-glucoside, beta-elemene, elemol, EO, eugenol, farnesene, farnesol, fat, fiber, geraniol, hesperidin, CIS-3-hexenyl-isovalerate, beta-humulene, iron, isobornyl-acetate, isomenthone, CIS-jasmone, limonene, linalool, luteolin, menthol, menthone, nedihydrocarveol, neryl-acetate, niacin, 3-octanol, 3-octyl-acetate, perillyl-alcohol, L-phellandrene, phosphorus, alpha-pinene, beta-pinene, piperitone, piperitenone-oxide, protein, pulegone, riboflavin, thiamin, valeric acid, water. (*FNF:* 18-19)

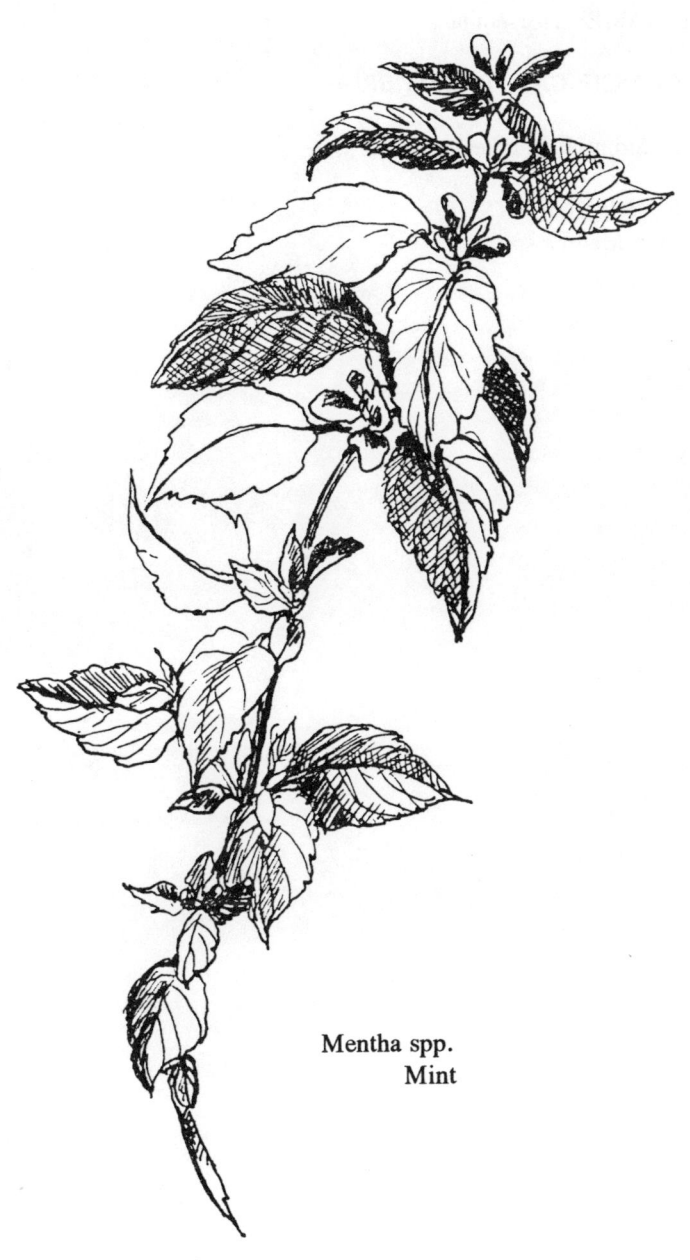

Mentha spp.
Mint

SCIENTIFIC NAME: Mentha spp.

LOCAL NAME: Horsemint

LEE'S CLASSIFICATION: MT SR A

USE(S): Stomach troubles

ACTIVE INGREDIENTS:
See the first Mentha spp.

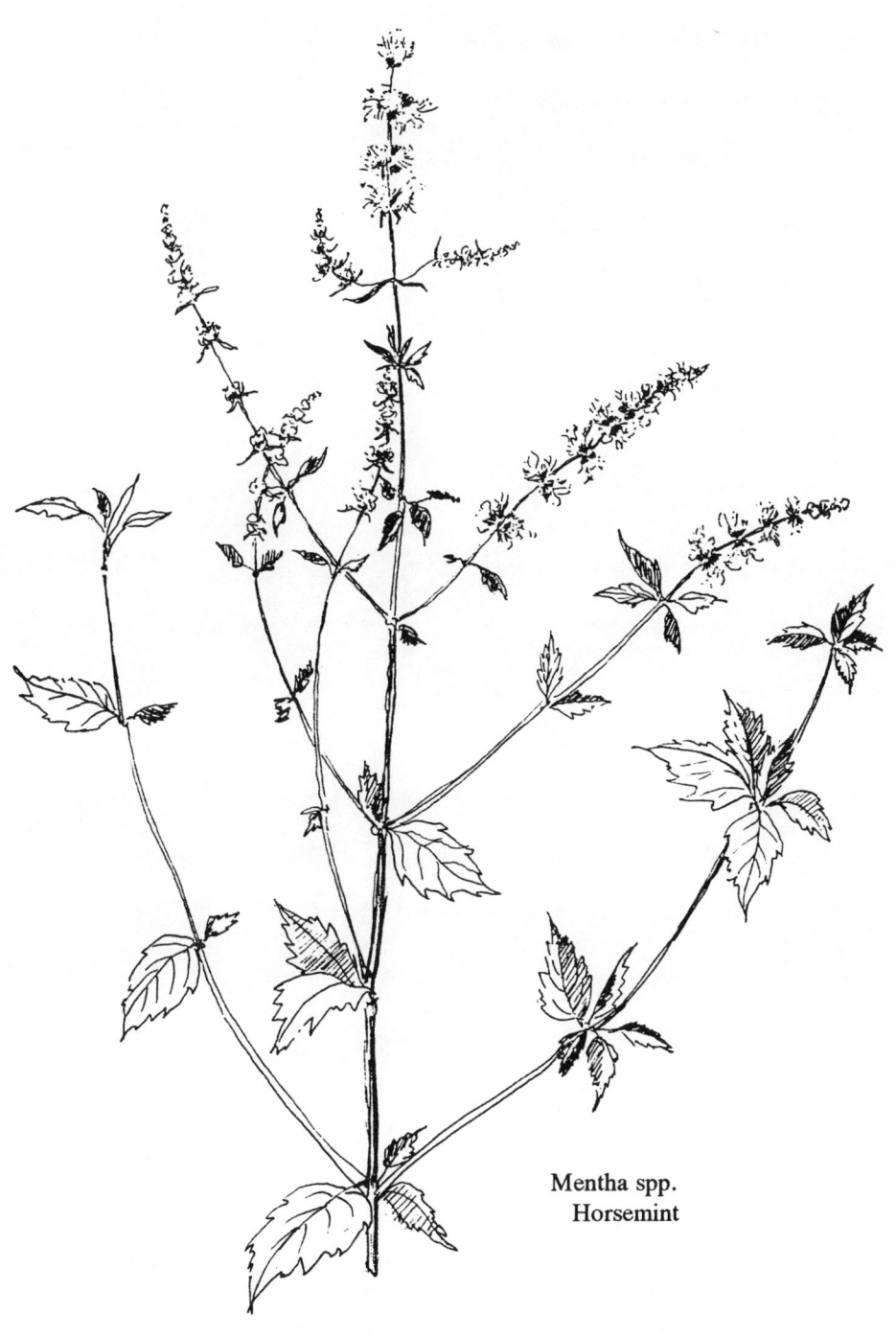

Mentha spp.
Horsemint

SCIENTIFIC NAME: Mentha spp.

LOCAL NAME: Housemint (Spearmint)

LEE'S CLASSIFICATION: ST MA VA

USE(S):   Stomach troubles

ACTIVE INGREDIENTS:
See the first Mentha spp.

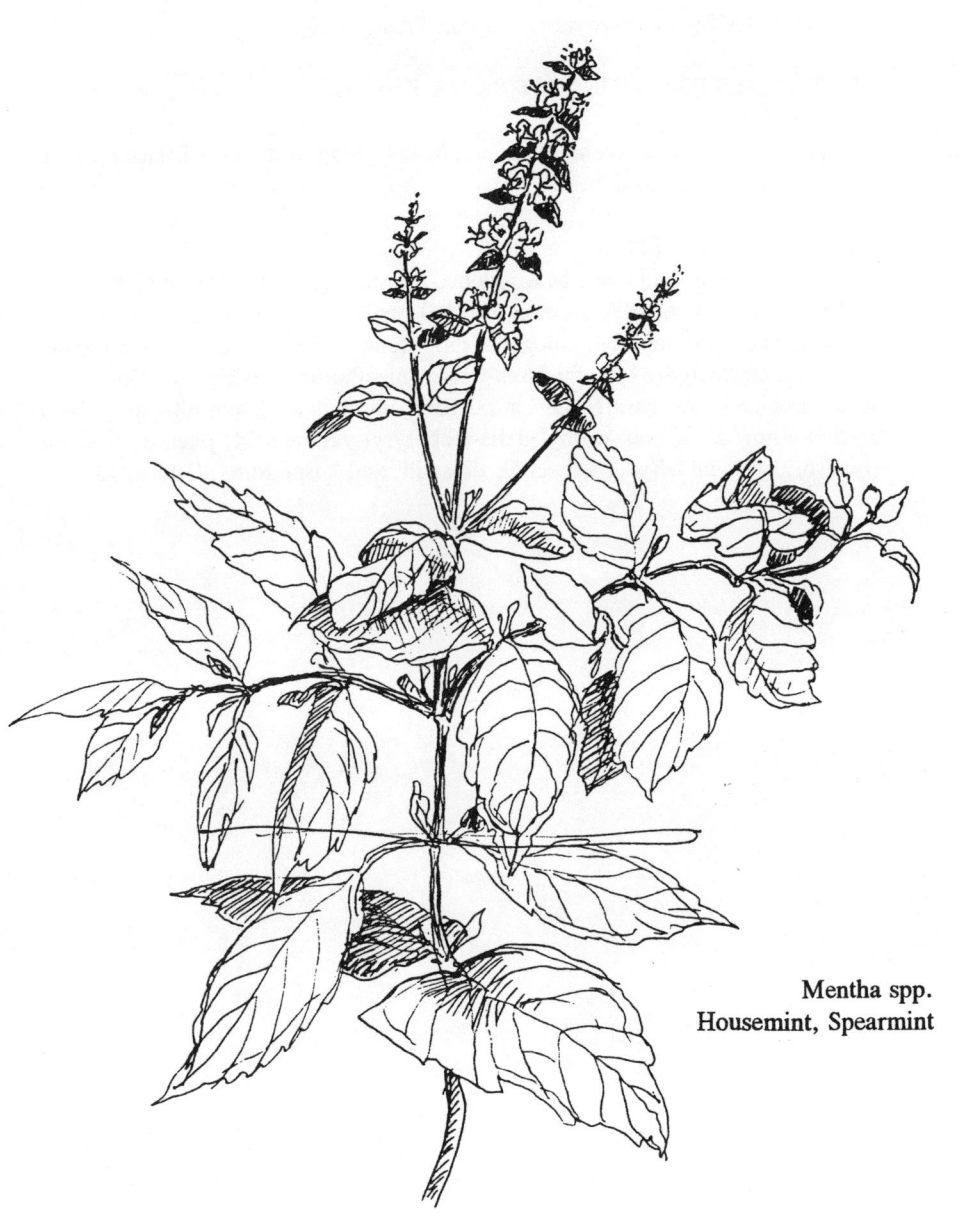

Mentha spp.
Housemint, Spearmint

SCIENTIFIC NAME: Mentha pulegium

LOCAL NAME: Pennyroyal (European Pennyroyal)

LEE'S CLASSIFICATION: MT SR VA Powerful

USE(S): Stomach problems, cancer, fevers, lung trouble, headache, colic, swelling, seed ticks

ACTIVE INGREDIENTS:
Essential oil: alpha-pinene, beta pinene, limonene, 3-octanone, p-cymene, 3-octylacetate, 3-octanol, 1-octen-3-ol, 3-methylcyclo-hexanone, menthone, isomenthone, isopuleg-one, pulegone, piperitone, cis- and trans-pulegone oxide, piperitenone, dehydroxymethofuran-oxide, menthofuran oxide, caryophyllene, beta-humulene, and paraffins. Lauric acid, myristic acid, palmitic acid, beta-methyl-adipic acid, beta-methyl-delta-isobutyryl-valeric acid, phenol, o-cresol, p-cresol, salicylaldehyde, eugeonal, diosmin, and hesperidin. (Duke: 308)

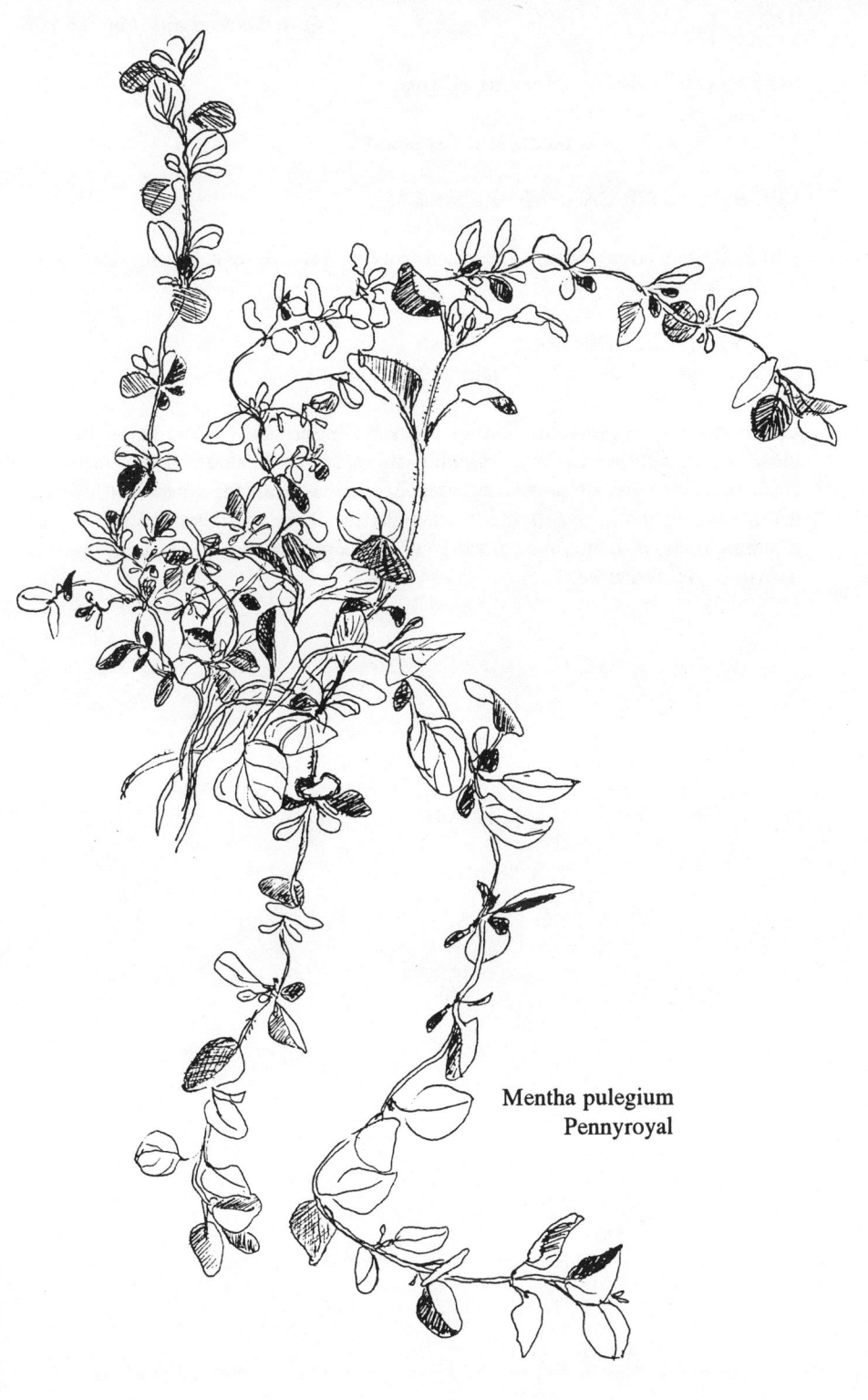

Mentha pulegium
Pennyroyal

SCIENTIFIC NAME: Monarda didyma

LOCAL NAME: Bee Balm, Red Bergamot

LEE'S CLASSIFICATION: ST MSR MA

USE(S): Menstrual cramps, stomach trouble, nervousness, carminative, gas, nausea

ACTIVE INGREDIENTS:
Natural source of thymol. (Duke: 279)

Essential oil with carvacol, thymol, cymene, bitterings. In the half-withered blossom: monardin; Leaves: essential oil contains linalool, linalyl acetate, limonene, ocemene, alpha-pinene, camphene, delta-3-carene, caravacrol, ursolic acid, beta-sitosterol, beta-carotene, pheophytine alpha and beta, and glucoside, didymin, linarine, flavonoids, gluco-genkwanin, genkwanin, naringenin, prunin, narirutin. (*Hagers:* 881)

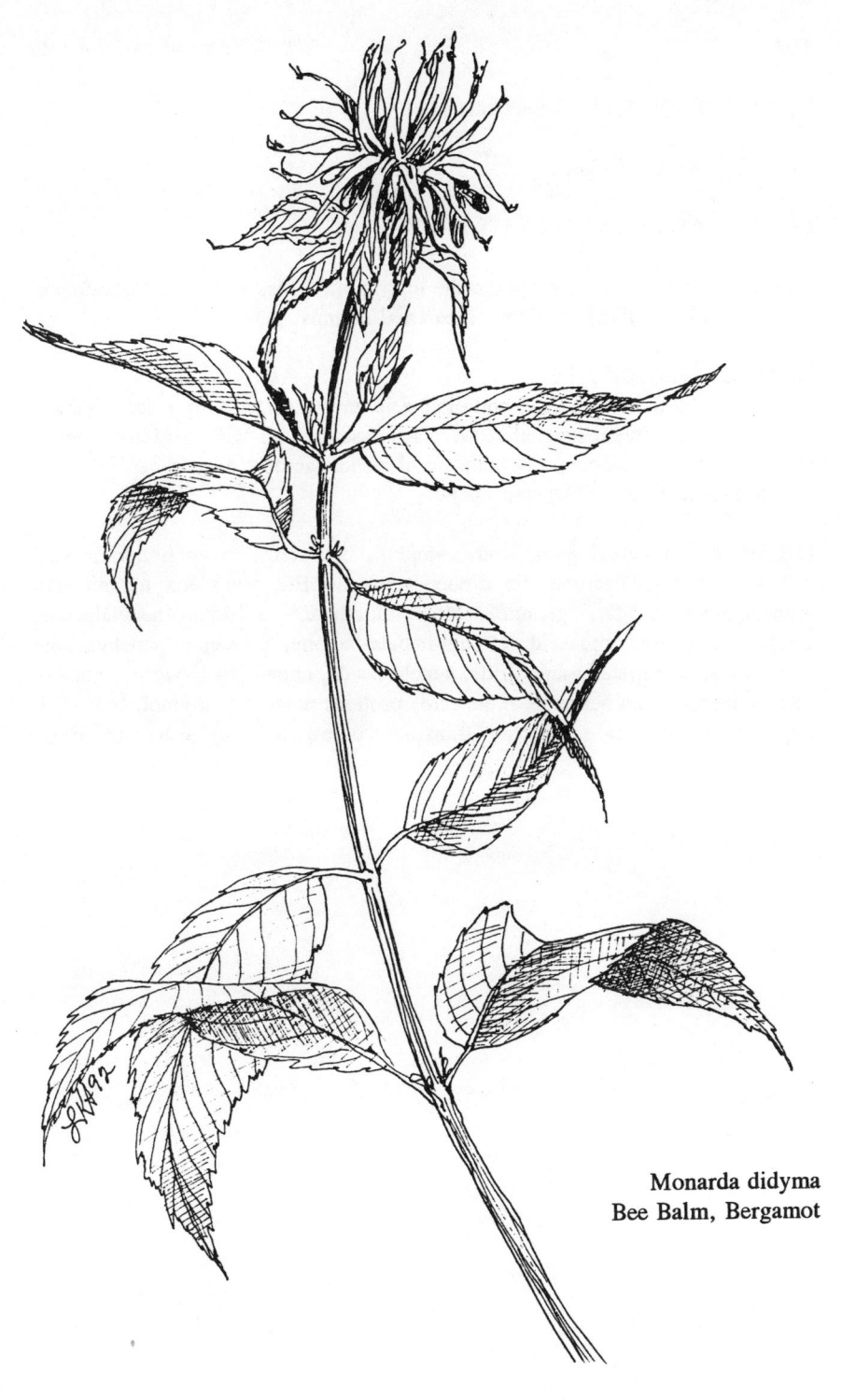

Monarda didyma
Bee Balm, Bergamot

SCIENTIFIC NAME: Nepeta cataria

LOCAL NAME: Catnip

LEE'S CLASSIFICATION: MT MR VA

USE(S): Colic, thrush, diaper rash, insomnia, colds, arthritis, chicken pox, hives, diarrhea, fever, menstrual cramps, gas

ACTIVE INGREDIENTS:
Dry seeds: linolenic, linoleic, and oleic acid and saturated fatty acids. Volatile oil, major constituent nepetalactone. An essential oil with geraniol (geranyl alcohol), citro-nellol, caryophyllene, nerol, nepetalactone, dihydronepeta-lacton, and epinepetalacton. (*Hagers:* 177)

(1R,5R,8S,9S)-deoxyloganic acid, camphor, carvacrol, caryophyllene, citral, 5,9,-dehydronepetalactone, dihydronepetalactone, EO, 5-epideoxyloganic acid, epinepetalactone, fat, geraniol, alpha-humulene, isodihydro-nepetalactone, linoleic acid, linolenic acid, methyl-nepeta-lactone, myrcene, nepetalactone, nepetalic acid, nepetalic-anhydride, nepetariaside, nepetoglucosylester, nepetol, CIS-ocimene, trans-ocimene, oleic acid, protein, pulegone, thymol, trans-CIS-nepetonic acid-methyl-ester, trans-trans-nepetonic acid-methyl-ester. (*FNF:* 43-44)

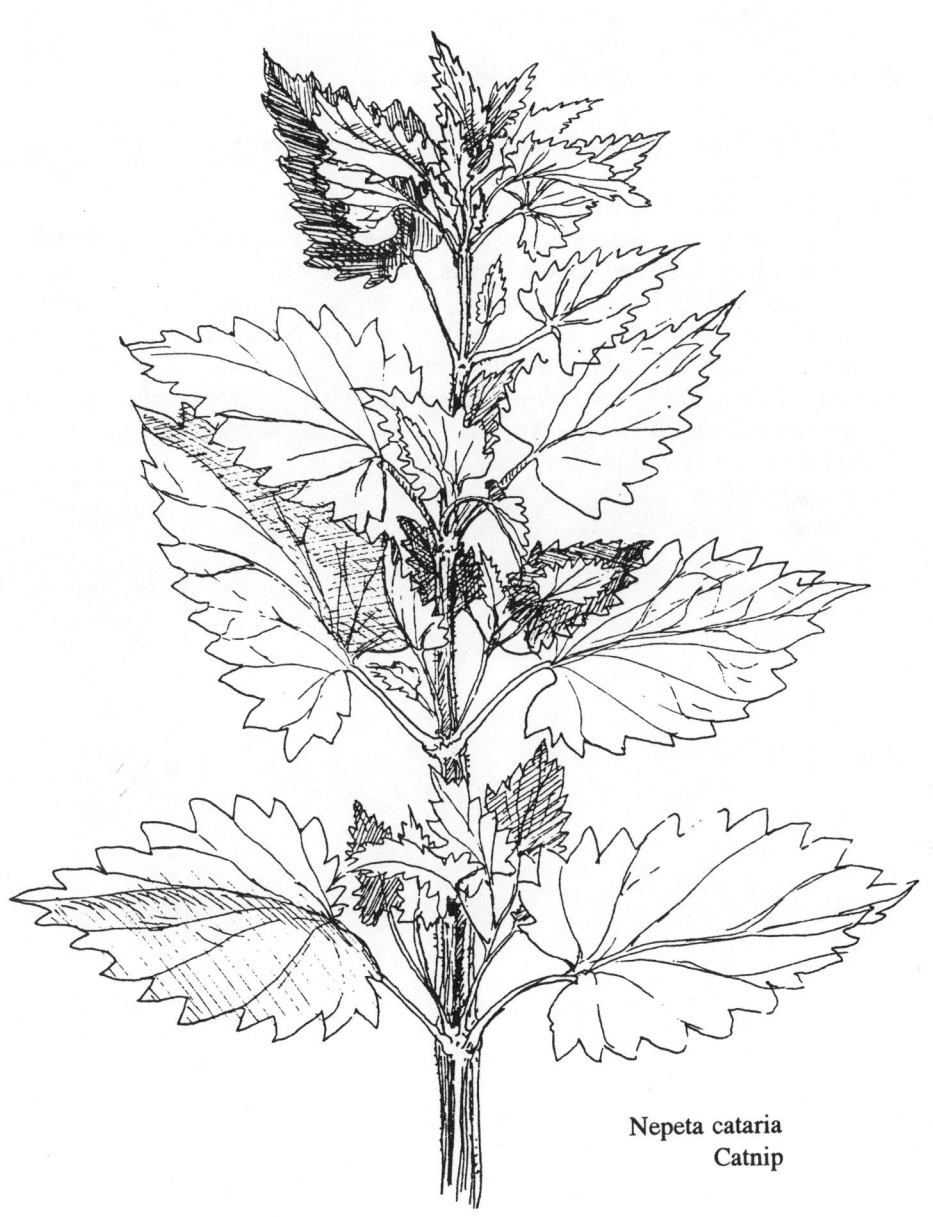

Nepeta cataria
Catnip

SCIENTIFIC NAME: Oenothera biennis

LOCAL NAME: Primrose (Evening)

LEE'S CLASSIFICATION: MT SR VA

USE(S): Tumors, coughs, colds, mental depression, rashes

ACTIVE INGREDIENTS:
Alanin, ammonia, alpha-amyrin, beta-amyrin, arginine, boron, aspartic acid, caffeic acid, calcium, carbohydrates, cellu-lose-lignin, citrostadieniol, O-coumaric acid, P-coumaric acid, delphinidin, digallic acid, ellagic acid, fat, fiber, gallic acid, kaempferol, alpha-linoleic acid, beta-linoleic acid, gamma-linolenic acid, magnesium, mucilage, neochloro-genic acid, oenotherin, oleic acid, palmitic acid, phloba-phene, phosphorus, phytosterol, potassium, protein, quer-cetin, resin, beta-sitosterol, stearic acid, tannin, alpha-tocopherol. (*FNF:* 48-50)

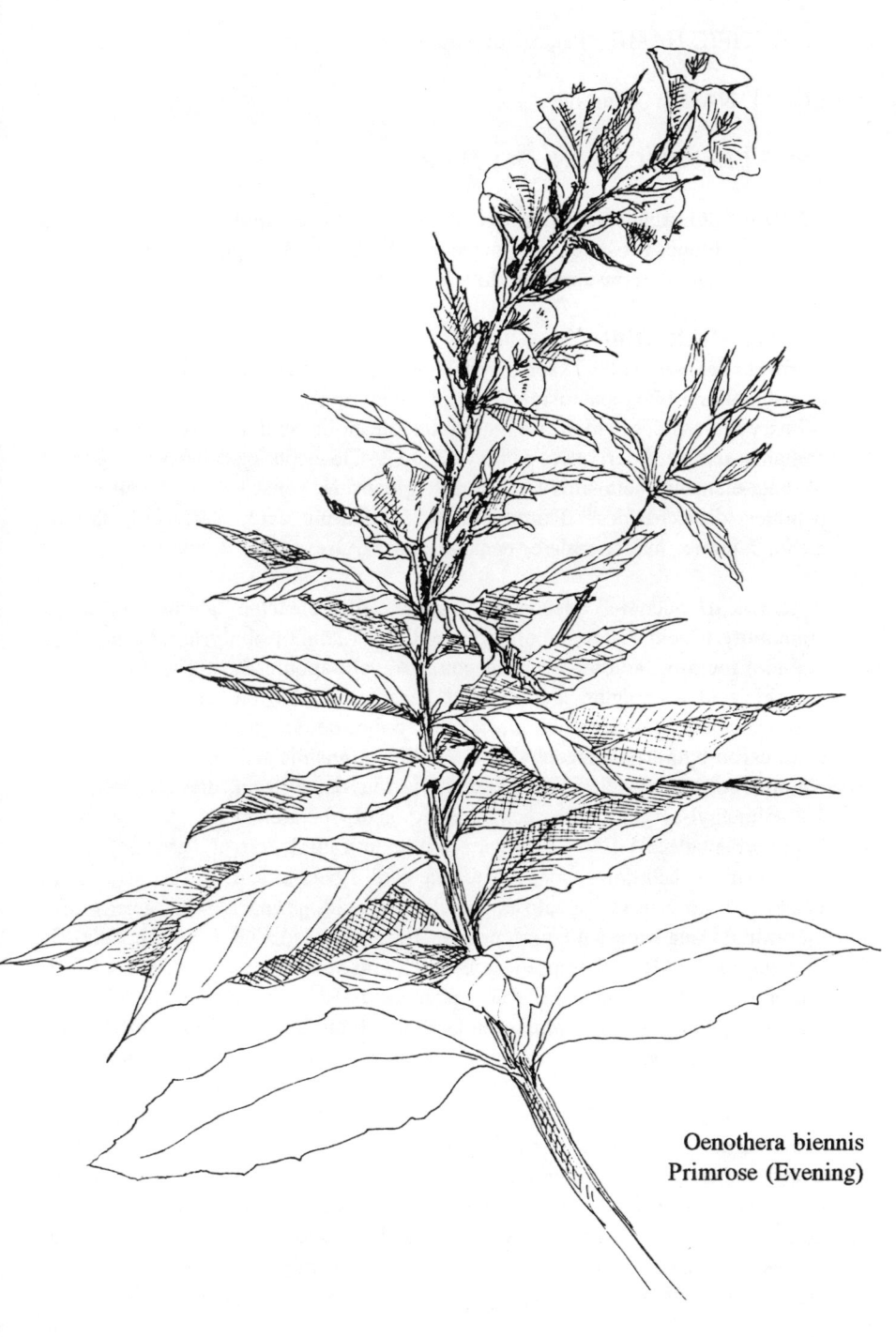

Oenothera biennis
Primrose (Evening)

SCIENTIFIC NAME: Panax quinquefolius

LOCAL NAME: Ginseng

LEE'S CLASSIFICATION: MT MR A

USE(S): Stomachaches, kidney and liver problems, diabetes, bad (unclean) blood, prostate gland problems, back and chest pains, low sex drive, nerves, consumption, low appetite

ACTIVE INGREDIENTS:
Herbage: panasenoside, a kaempferd-3-glucogalactoside, kaempferol and trifolin and something like panaxoside C; Roots: contain a complex array of saponins, primary glycosides which are based on oleanolic acid or dammarol. Also contains: acetylene derivative panaxynol, a 1,9-CIS-hepta-decadiene-4,6,-diyn-3-ol, beta-elemene, beta-sitos-terol and its glucoside, panacene, a pyrrolidine, 5-peptides, disaccharides. Pantothenic acid, nicotinic acid, oleic acid, choline, citric, fumaric, malic, maleic, panaxic, and tartaric acids. (Duke: 341)

Acetic acid, adenine, adenosine, alanine, alloisoleucine, aluminum, alpha-aminobutyric acid, beta-aminobutyric acid, beta-aminoisobutyric acid, amylase, arabinofuranose, arabinose, arasaponin-A, arasaponin-B, arginine, arsenic, ascorbic acid, asparagine, aspartic acid, benzoic acid, bicyclogermacrene, biotin, boron, N-butyric acid, calcium, calcium-polyuronide, campesterol, N-caproic acid, carbo-hydrates, caryophyllene, choline, cinnamic acid, citric acid, cobalt, colonin, copper, cysteic acid, cysteine, cystine, daucosterin, diastase, dextrose, 1,3,-dimethyl-acrylic acid, echinocystic acid, beta-elemene, 9,10-epoxy-3-hydroxyheptadeca-1-EN-4,6,-diyne, escin, estradiol, estrol, estrone, ethyl-machaerinate, beta-farnesene, fat, ferulic acid, fiber, folic acid, formic acid, D-fructose, fumaric-acid, galactose, galacturonic acid, germacrene-D, germanium, ginsenin, ginsenoside-R-O, ginsenoside-RB, ginsenoside-RB-1, ginsenoside-RB-2, ginsenoside-RB-4, ginsenoside-RC, ginseno-side-RD, ginsenoside-RE, ginsenoside-RF, ginsenoside-RG, ginsenoside-RG-1, ginsenoside-RG-2, D-glucose, glucuronic acid, glucuronolactone, glutamic acid, glutamose, glutaric acid, glycine, guanidine, guanine heptadeca-1-EN-4,6-diyn-3,9-diol, 1,9-CIS,heptadecadiene-1,6-diyn-3-OL, 9-CIS,hepta-decadiene-4,6-diyn-3-OL, 1-heptadecaene-4,6-diyn-3,8,10-triol, 1-heptadecaene-4,6-diyn-3,8-diol, histidine, alpha-humulene, beta-humulene, hydroxycholine, P-hydroxycinnamic acid, 3-hydroxy-5-methyl-gamma-pyrone, hydroxyproline, iodine, iron, isobutyric acid, isoleucine, isovaleric acid, kaempferol, kaempferol-3-glucogalactoside, ketoglutaric acid, leucine, levulose, linoleic acid, linolenic acid, lysine, magnesium, maleic acid, malic acid, malonic acid, maltol, maltose, manganese, methionine, methyl-butyricacid, molybdenum, O-monomethylaminobenzoicacid,

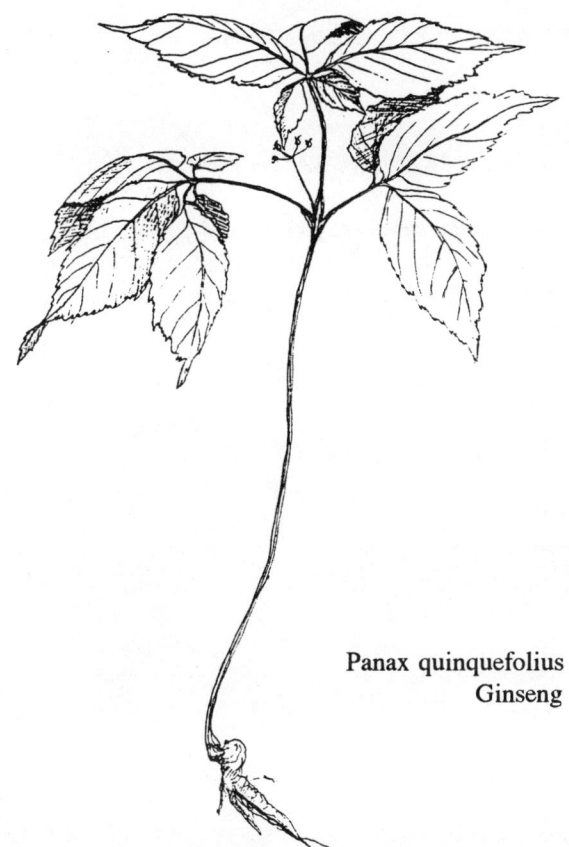

Panax quinquefolius
Ginseng

alpha-neoclovene, beta-neoclovene, niacin, nicotinic acid, nitrogen, nona-cosane, 1-octacosanol, oleanolic acid, oleic acid, palmitic acid, panacen, panaquilon, alpha-panasinsene, beta-pana-sinsene, panax acid, panacen, panaquilon, alpha-panasinsene, beta-panasinsene, panax acid, panaxadiol, panaxasapogenin, panaxasapogenol, panaxatriol, panaxic acid, panaxin, panaxoside-A, panaxoside-B, panaxoside-C, panaxoside-D, panaxoside-E, panaxoside-F, panaxydiol, panaxynol, panto-thenic acid, pectin, petroselinic acid, petroselaidic acid, phenolase, phenylalanine, phosphorus, potassium, proline, propionic acid, prostisol, protein, protopanaxadion, proto-panaxatriol, alpha-pyrrolidone, pyruvic-acid, raffinose, resin, L-rhamnose, riboflavin, saccharose, saikosaponin-A, saikosaponin-B, salicylic acid, beta-santalene, saponin, alpha-selinene, beta-selinene, gamma-selinene, serine, silicon, beta-sitosterol, beta-sitosterol-glycoside, sodium, starch, stearic acid, stigmasterol, strontium, succinic acid, sucrose, sulfur, tannin, tartaric acid, tenuifolic acid, threonine, tiglic acid, tyrosine, uracil, uridine, uronic acid, N-valeric acid, valine, vanadium, vanillic acid, vitamin B-12, D-xylose, zinc. (*FNF:* 63-66)

SCIENTIFIC NAME: Phoradendron serotinum

LOCAL NAME: Mistletoe

LEE'S CLASSIFICATION: ST SR VA Powerful

USE(S): Abortifacient (used only in the old days)

ACTIVE INGREDIENTS:
Beta-phenylethylamine, tyramine. (Duke: 364)

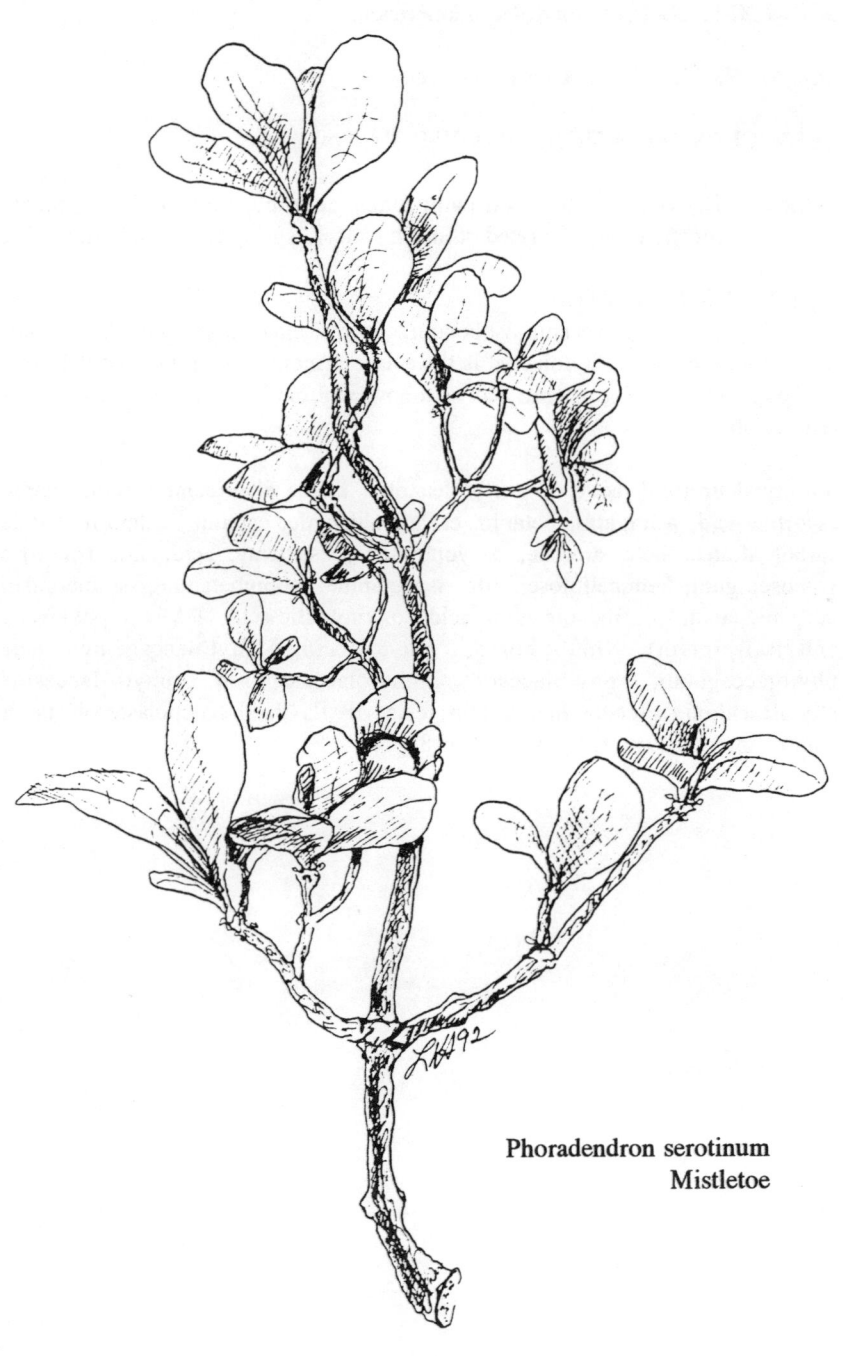

Phoradendron serotinum
Mistletoe

SCIENTIFIC NAME: Phytolacca americana

LOCAL NAME: Poke Root (Pokeweed)

LEE'S CLASSIFICATION: VST VSR VA Powerful

USE(S): Thyroid trouble, chest pain, fungal skin infections, arthritis, ulcers, constipation, ulcerated stomach cancer, spring tonic, impetigo, cysts

ACTIVE INGREDIENTS:
Caryophyllene, phytolaccanin, isobetanine, isoprebetanine, and prebetanine; salts of phytolaccic acid. Phytolaccin is the active principle in all parts of the plant. A sapogenin, phytolaccagenin acts as a powerful molluscicide and parasiticide. (Duke: 367)

3-acetylaleurotolic acid, 3-acetyloleanolic acid, americanin, anthocyanin, ascorbic acid, astragalin, betanin, caffeic-aldehyde, calcium, calcium-oxalate, carbohydrates, beta-carotene, caryophyllene, esculentic acid, fat, fruc-tose, glucose, gum, hemicellulose, iron, isobetanine, isoprebetanine, isoquercitrin, jaligonic acid, niacin, oleanolic-acid, oxymyristic-acid, PAP (=pokeweed-antiviral-protein), phosphorus, phytolaccin, phytolaccagenic acid, phytolaccagenin, phytolaccanin, phytolaccasaponin, phyto-laccaside, phytolaccatoxin, prebetanine, protein, resin, riboflavin, alpha-spinasterol, starch, tannin, thiamin, water, xylose. (*FNF:*83-84)

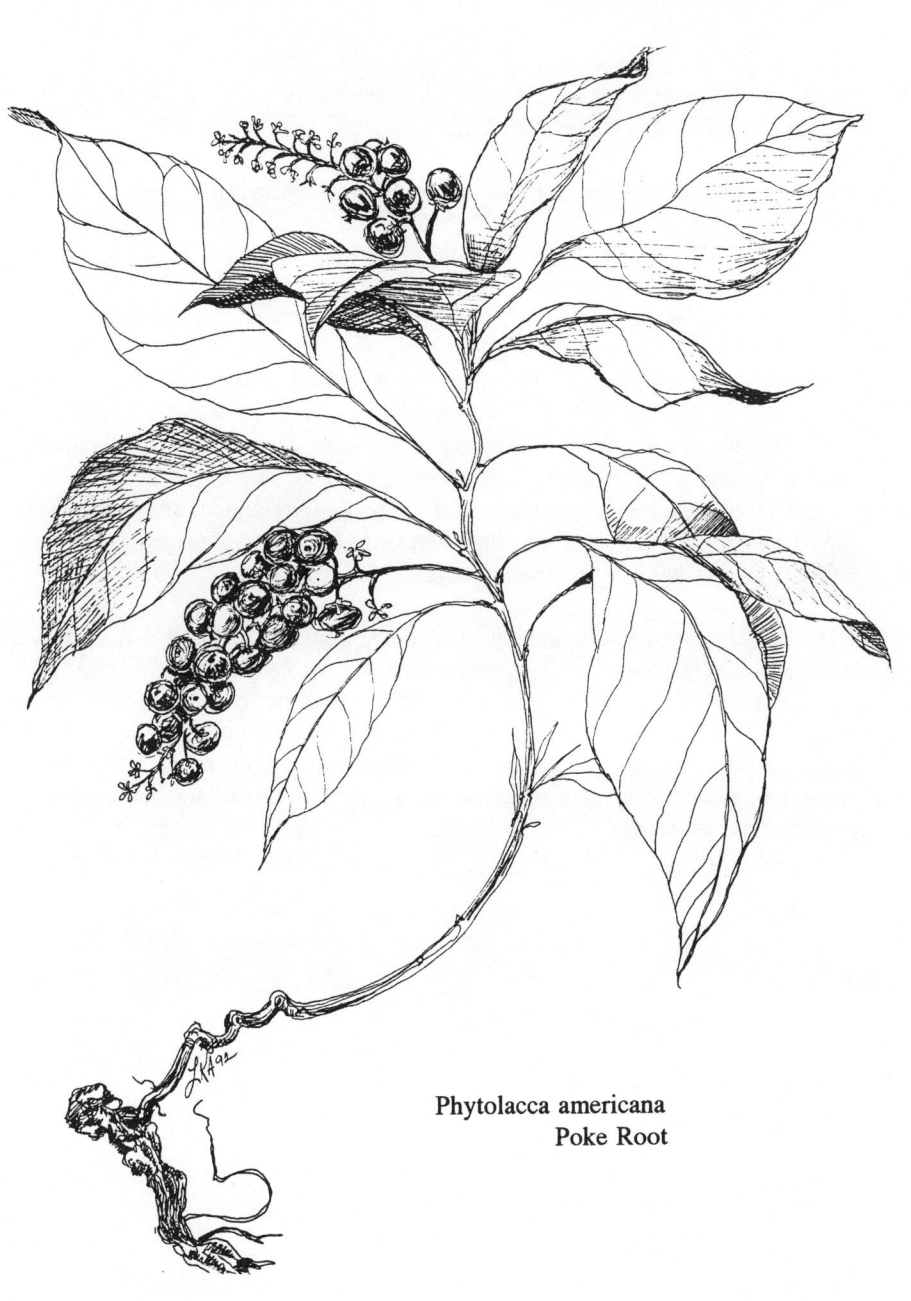

Phytolacca americana
Poke Root

SCIENTIFIC NAME: Pinus strobus

LOCAL NAME: White Pine Top (Eastern White Pine)

LEE'S CLASSIFICATION: MT MR A

USE(S): Fevers, pneumonia, flu, colds, measles, whooping cough, soreness in the chest

ACTIVE INGREDIENTS:
Several species exude oleoresins (turpentine). (*Wealth of Ind.*: 64-65)

Seeds may yield turpentine. Bark may contain tannin. (Watt and Breyer: 843)

Leucocyanidin; resin acid in the resin: abietic acid, pimar, levopimaric, sandaracopimaric, isopimaric, dehydroabietic, and neoabietic acid; Kernel: pinosylvin, pinosylvin-mono-methyl ester, its dihydro compound pinocembrin, pinobanksin, chrysin, pinostrobin, techtochrysin; Bark: diterpenes, strobol, strobal, monoxide, cis- and trans-abienol. (*Hagers:* 692)

CIS-abienol, trans-abienol, abietic acid, amino acids, anticopalic acid, chrysin, coniferin, coniferyl-alcohol, cryptostrocin, dehydroabietic acid, elliotic acid, fat, isopimaric acid, laevopimaric acid, leucocyanidin, manoy-oxide, 3-beta-methoxy-14-serraten-21-ON, mucilage, neoabietinic acid, nucleic acids, palustric acid, pimaric acid, pinobanksin, pinocembrin, pinostrobin, pinosylvin-monomethyl-ester, sandaracopimaric acid, strobal, strobinic acid, strobol, strobopinin, tectochrysin. (*FNF:* 91-92)

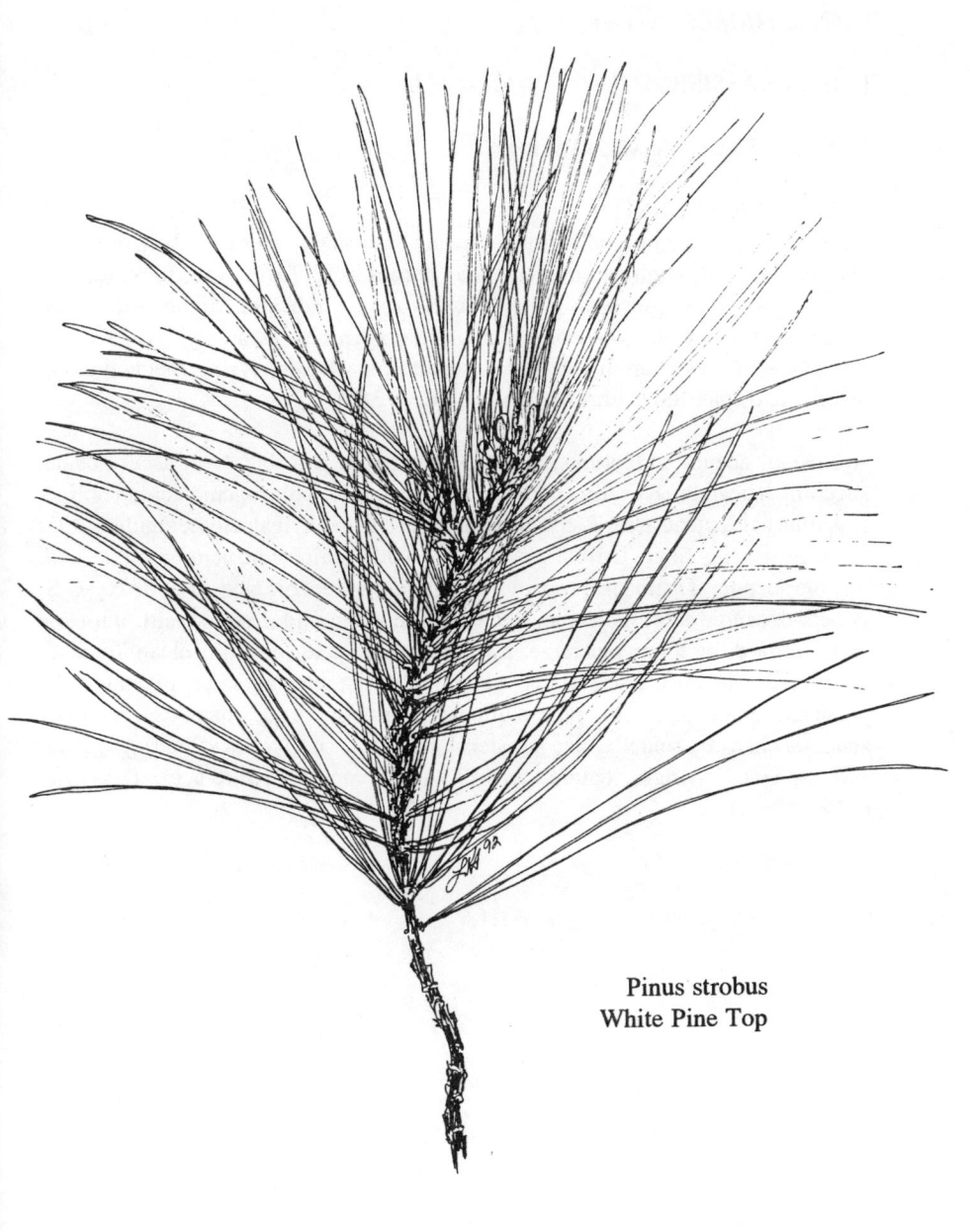

Pinus strobus
White Pine Top

SCIENTIFIC NAME: Plantago major

LOCAL NAME: Plantain

LEE'S CLASSIFICATION: ___ MR MA

USE(S): Sores, bruises, swelling

ACTIVE INGREDIENTS:
Aucubin, resin, tannin, allantoin, adenine, baicalein, baicalin, benzoic acid, chlorogenic acid, choline, cinnamic acid, ferulic acid, L-fructose, fumaric acid, gentisic acid, D-glucose, P-hydroxybenzoic, indicain, lignoceric acid, neochlorogenic acid, oleanolic acid, plantagonine, planteose, saccharose, salicylic acid, scutellarein, sitosterol, sorbitol, stachyose, syringicacid, tyrosol, ursolic acid, vanillic acid, D-xylose. (Duke: 386)

Acetoside, adenine, alkaloids, allantoin, apigenin, ascorbic acid, asperuloside, aucubin, baicalein, baicalin, benzoic acid, catalpol, chlorogenic acid, choline, cinnamic acid, citric acid, P-coumaric acid, D1-0-methylgalactose, emulsin, EO, fat, ferulic acid, fiber, L-fructose, fumaric acid, geniposidic acid, gentisic acid, glucoraphenine, D-glucose, hispidulin, P-hydroxybenzoic acid, 9-hydroxy-CIS-H-octa-decanoic acid, indicaine, invertin, lignoceric acid, linoleic acid, linolenic acid, loliolid, luteolin, mucilage, neochlorogenic acid, nepetin, oleanolic acid, oleic acid, phenolcarbonic acids, plantagic acids, plantagonine, plantagoside, plantease, planteolic acid, potassium-salis, protein, resin, rhamnose, salicylic acid, saccharose, scutellarein, sitosterol, sorbitol, succinic acid, syringic acid, sulforaphene, syringin, tannin, tyrosol, ursolic acid, vanillic acid, D-xylose. (*FNF:* 103-4)

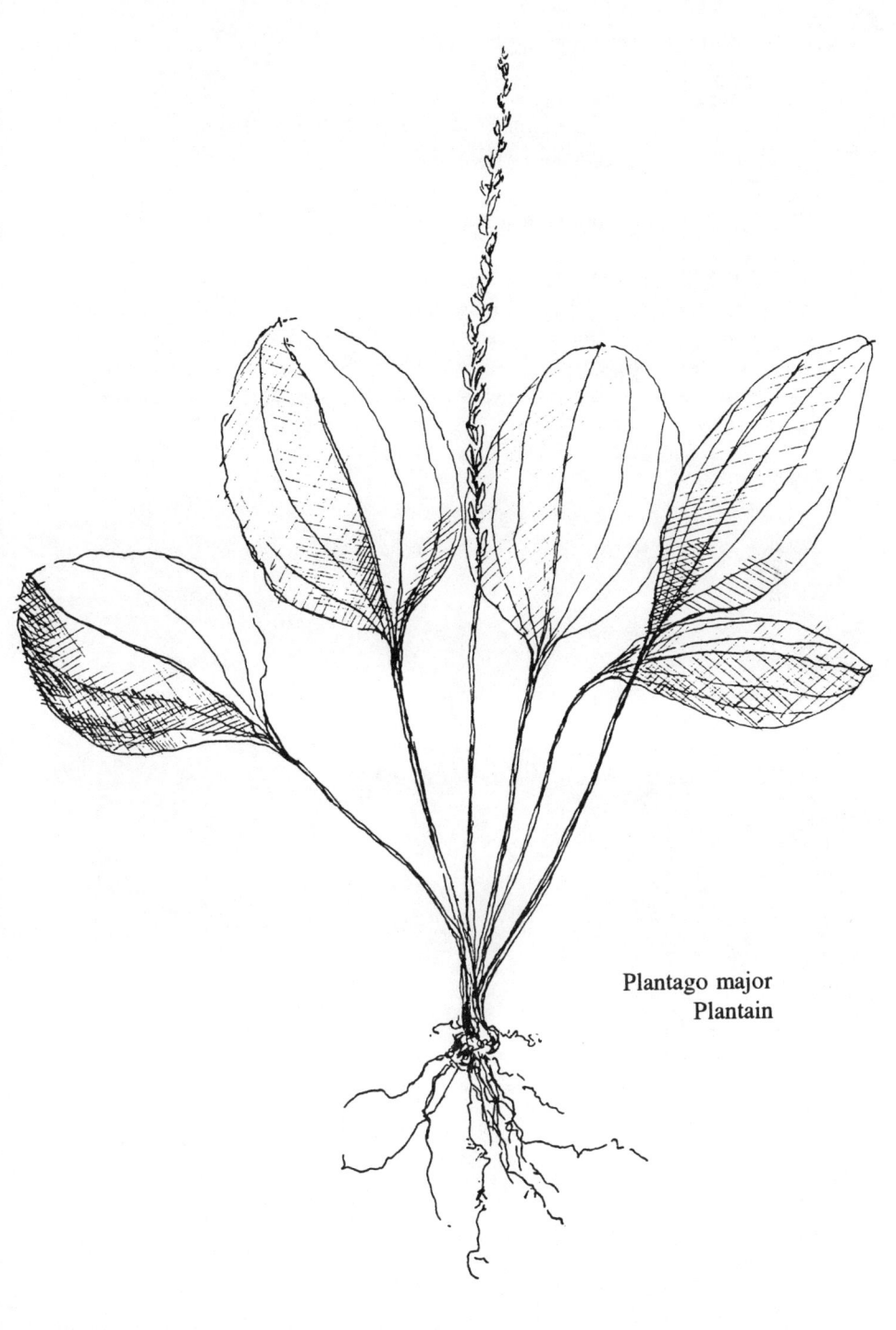

Plantago major
Plantain

SCIENTIFIC NAME: Podophyllum peltatum

LOCAL NAME: Mayapple

LEE'S CLASSIFICATION: ST SR VA

USE(S): Menstrual problems

ACTIVE INGREDIENTS:
Astragalin, berberine, dehydropodophyllotoxin, gallic acid, isorhamnetin, lignan-k, lignan-m, podophyllotoxin, podo-phyllin, podophyllic acid, picropodophyllin, alpha-peltatin, beta-peltatin. Several flavonoids: castragalin, isorham-netin, kaempferol, kaempferol-3-glucoside, quercetin, quer-cetin-3-galactoside, resin. (*FNF:* 107)

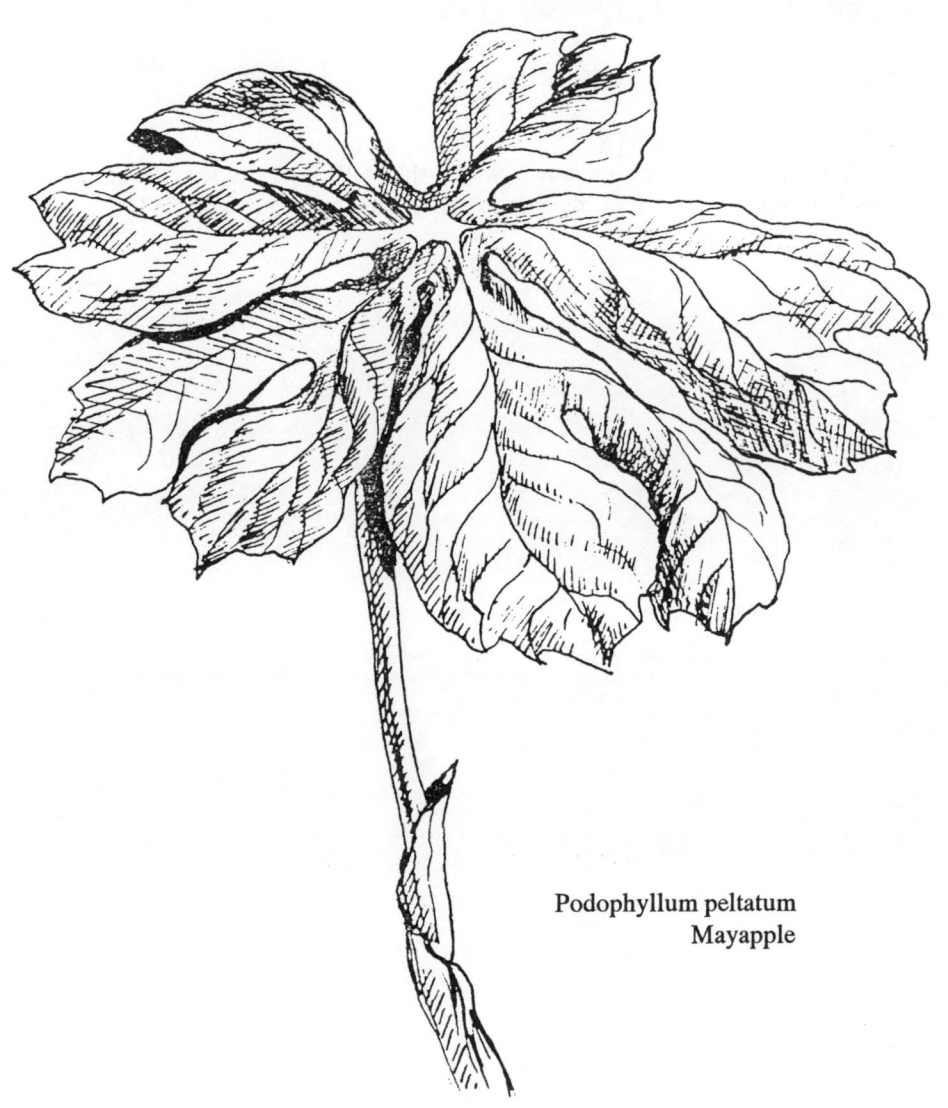

Podophyllum peltatum
Mayapple

SCIENTIFIC NAME: Polygonum pennsylvanica

LOCAL NAME: Pigweed, Pinkweed

LEE'S CLASSIFICATION: MT SR VA

USE(S): Stomach cancer, diabetes

ACTIVE INGREDIENTS:
Other species of polygonum contain the following toxins: gallic acid, hydrocyanic acid, indican, quercetin, rutin, tannic acid. (Duke: 563)

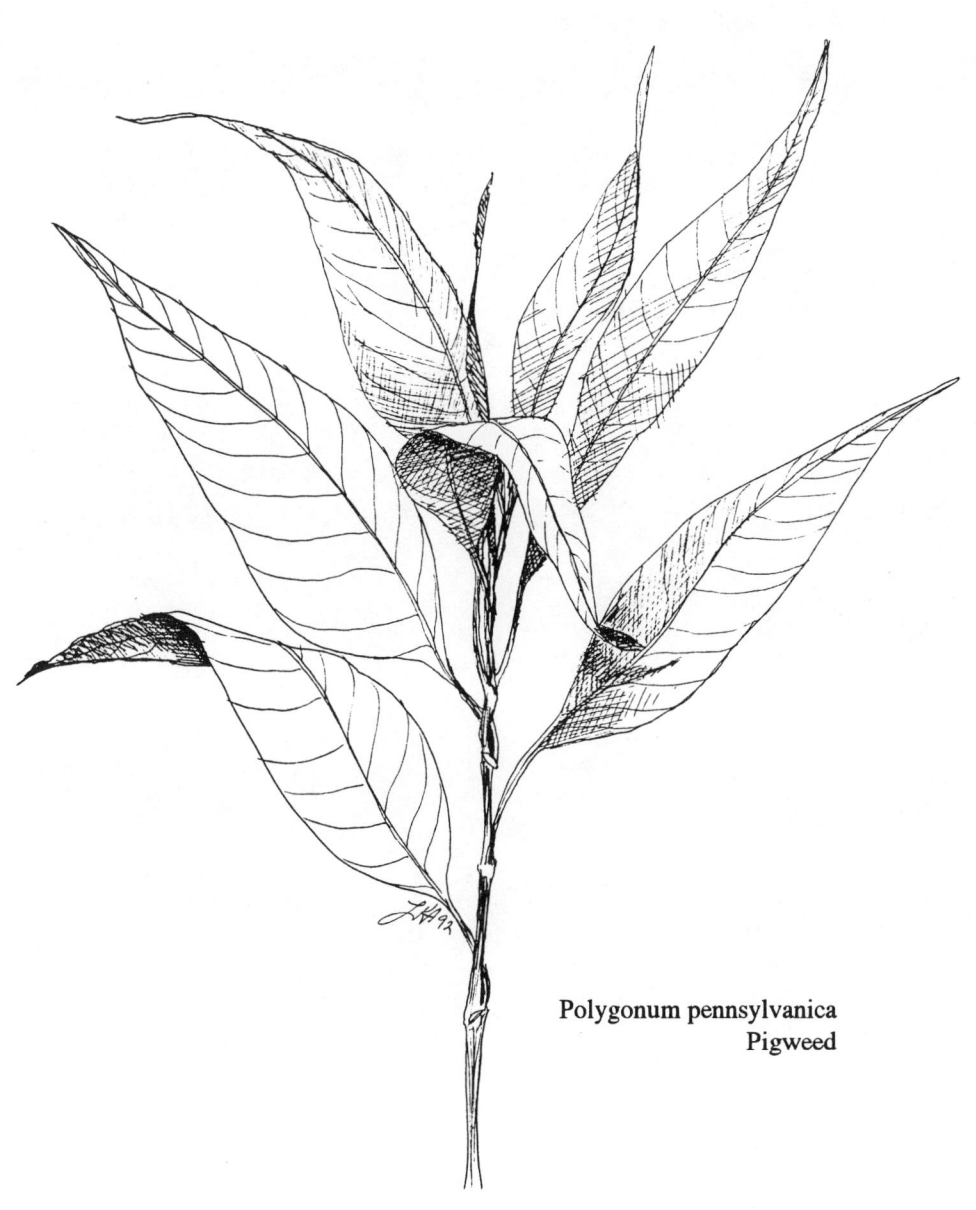

Polygonum pennsylvanica
Pigweed

SCIENTIFIC NAME: Polymnia uvedalia

LOCAL NAME: Bear's Foot

LEE'S CLASSIFICATION: MT MS A

USE(S): Cold, fever, stomach and kidney problems, heart problems, diabetes, arthritis, prostate gland problems, swelling, dandruff, irritation in the eye, loss of appetite

ACTIVE INGREDIENTS:
No references found for this herb.

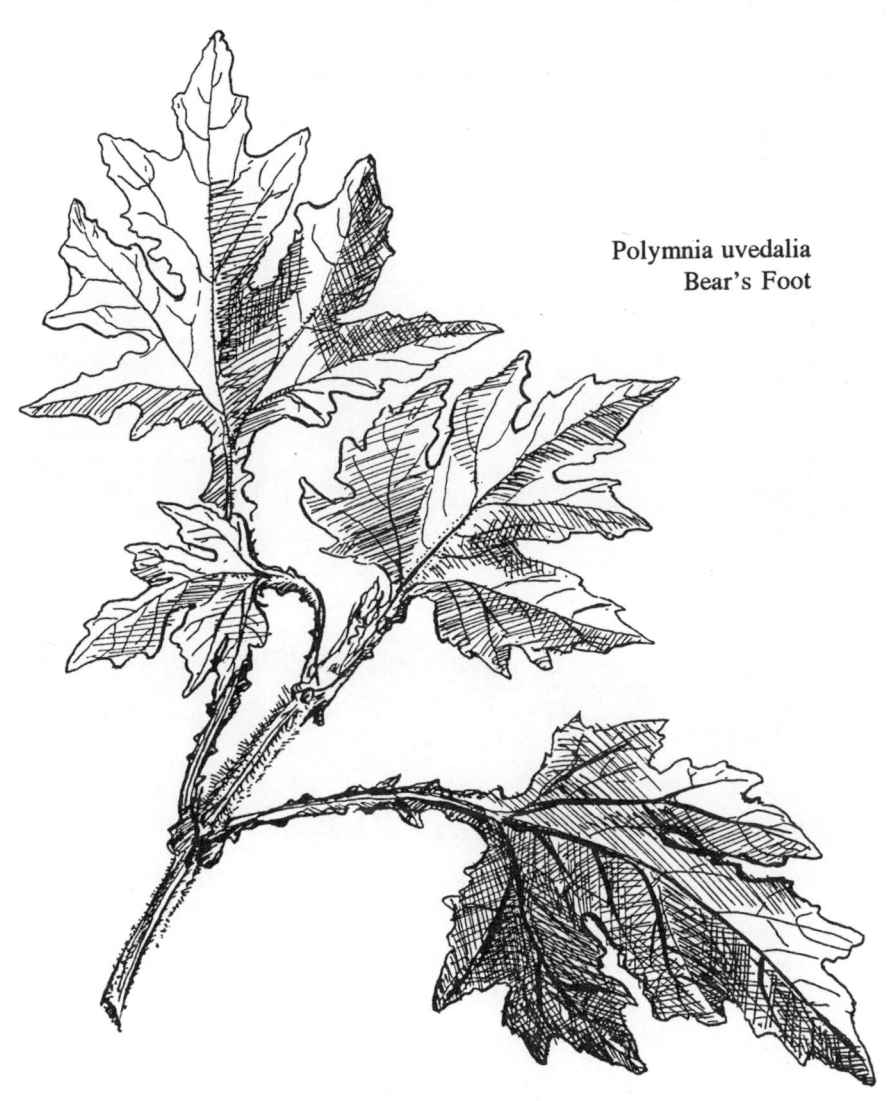

Polymnia uvedalia
Bear's Foot

SCIENTIFIC NAME: Polystichum acrostichoides

LOCAL NAME: Male Fern (Christmas)

LEE'S CLASSIFICATION: ST VSR VA

USE(S):   Worms

ACTIVE INGREDIENTS:
No references found for this herb.

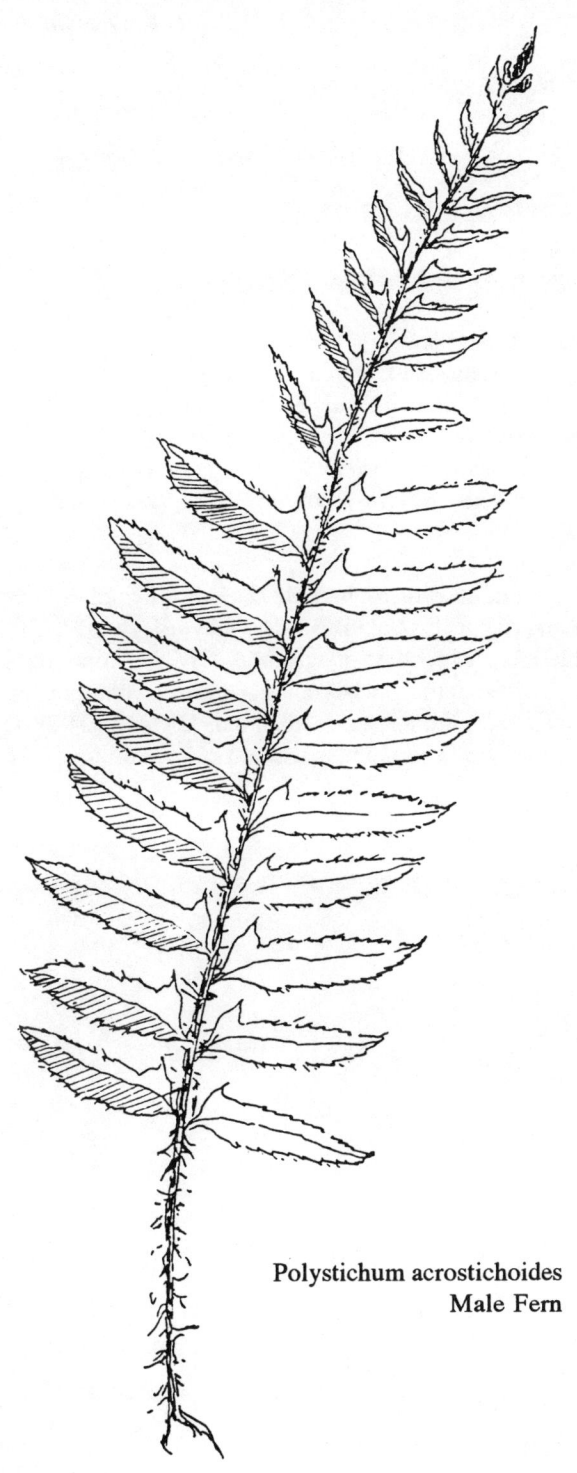

Polystichum acrostichoides
Male Fern

SCIENTIFIC NAME: Prunus serotina

LOCAL NAME: Wild Cherry (Black Cherry)

LEE'S CLASSIFICATION: ST SR A

USE(S): Coughs, colds, hoarseness, indigestion

ACTIVE INGREDIENTS:
Bark contains the cyanogenetic glycoside prunasin and the enzyme prunase (or emulsin), which yields an hydrolysis HCN. (Duke: 376)

Prunasin, emulsin, eudesmic acid, p-coumaric acid, scopoletin, tanin. The amount of prussic acid changes according to the season and age of the bark. (*Hagers:* 950)

Acetylcholine, aluminum, ash, barium, boron, calcium, chromium, cobalt, copper, P-coumaric acid, 2-alpha-3-alpha-dihydroxyurs-12-EN-28-OIC acid, emulsin, eudesmic acid, beta-glycosidase, HCN, iron, lanthanum, lead, magnesium, molybdenum, neodymium, nickle, phosphorus, potassium, scopoletin, silver, strontium, tannin, titanium, URS-12-EN-28-AL-3-beta-OL, ursolic acid, vanadium, ytterbium, yttrium, zinc, zirconium. (*FNF:* 126-27)

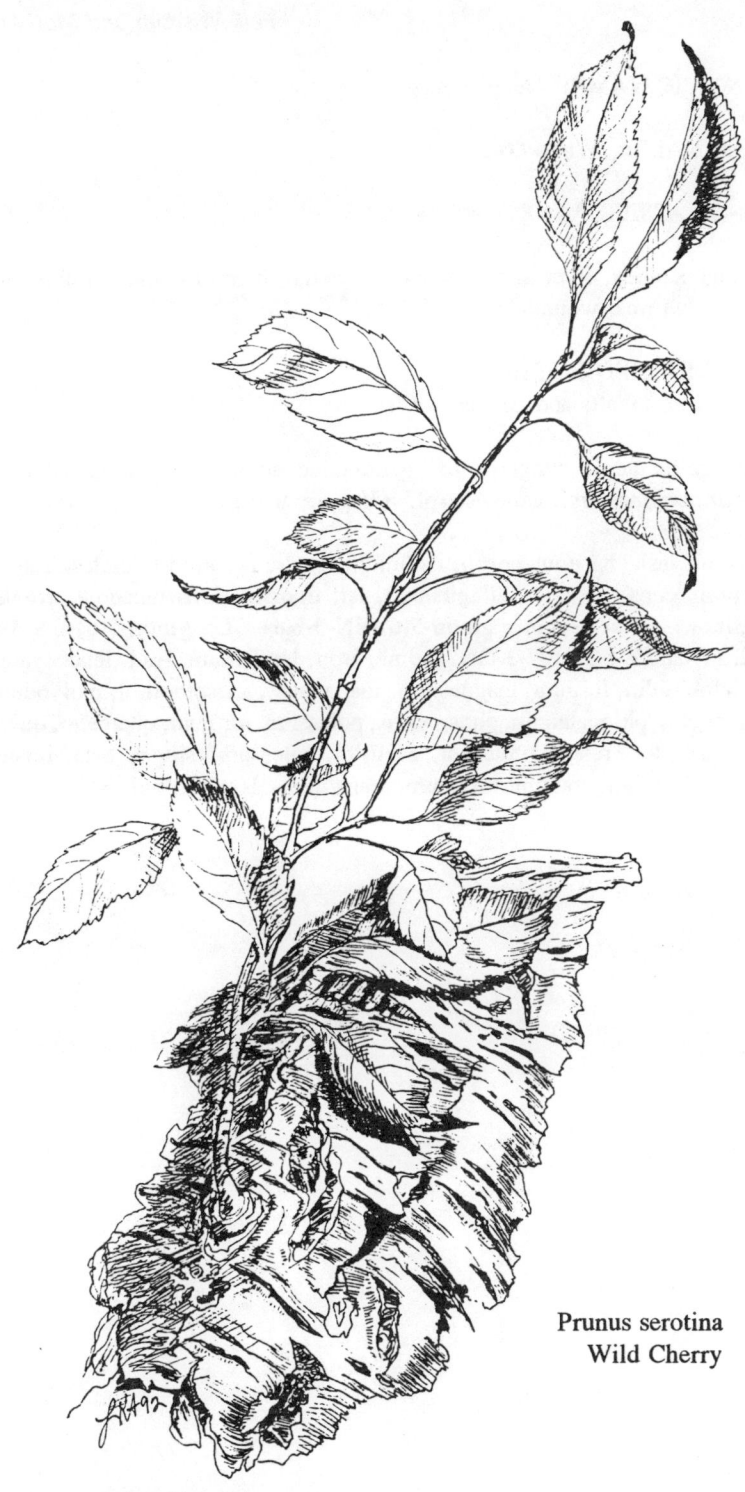

Prunus serotina
Wild Cherry

SCIENTIFIC NAME: Quercus alba

LOCAL NAME: White Oak Bark

LEE'S CLASSIFICATION: ST SR A

USE(S): Kidney, liver and stomach problems; hemorrhoids; varicose veins; worms; wounds

ACTIVE INGREDIENTS:
Bark: tannin. (Watts and Breyer: 439)

Wood: gallic acid, ellagic acid, gallotannic acid, camphenylaldehyde, B-sitosterin, stigmasterol, campesterol. (*Hagers:* 1012)

Aluminum, ash, barium, boron, cadmium, calcium, carbo-hydrates, catechin, chromium, cobalt, copper, ellagitannin, fat, fluorine, 3-friedelanone, friedelin, friedelinol, gallocatechin, glutin-5(6)-EN-3-beta-OL, glutin-5(6)-EN-3-ON, 2,hydroxydammar-24-EN-3-ON, iodine, iron, lanthanum, lead, leucocyanidin, leucodelphinidin, lithium, magnesium, manganese, mesoinolitol, molybdenum, nickel, pectin, phlobatannin, phosphorus, potassium, protein, quercetin, quercin, L-(+)-quercitol, resin, rubidium, scyllitol, selenium, silver, beta-sitosterol, sodium, strontium, tannin, titanium, vanadium, L-viburnitol, yttrium, zinc. (*FNF:* 146-47)

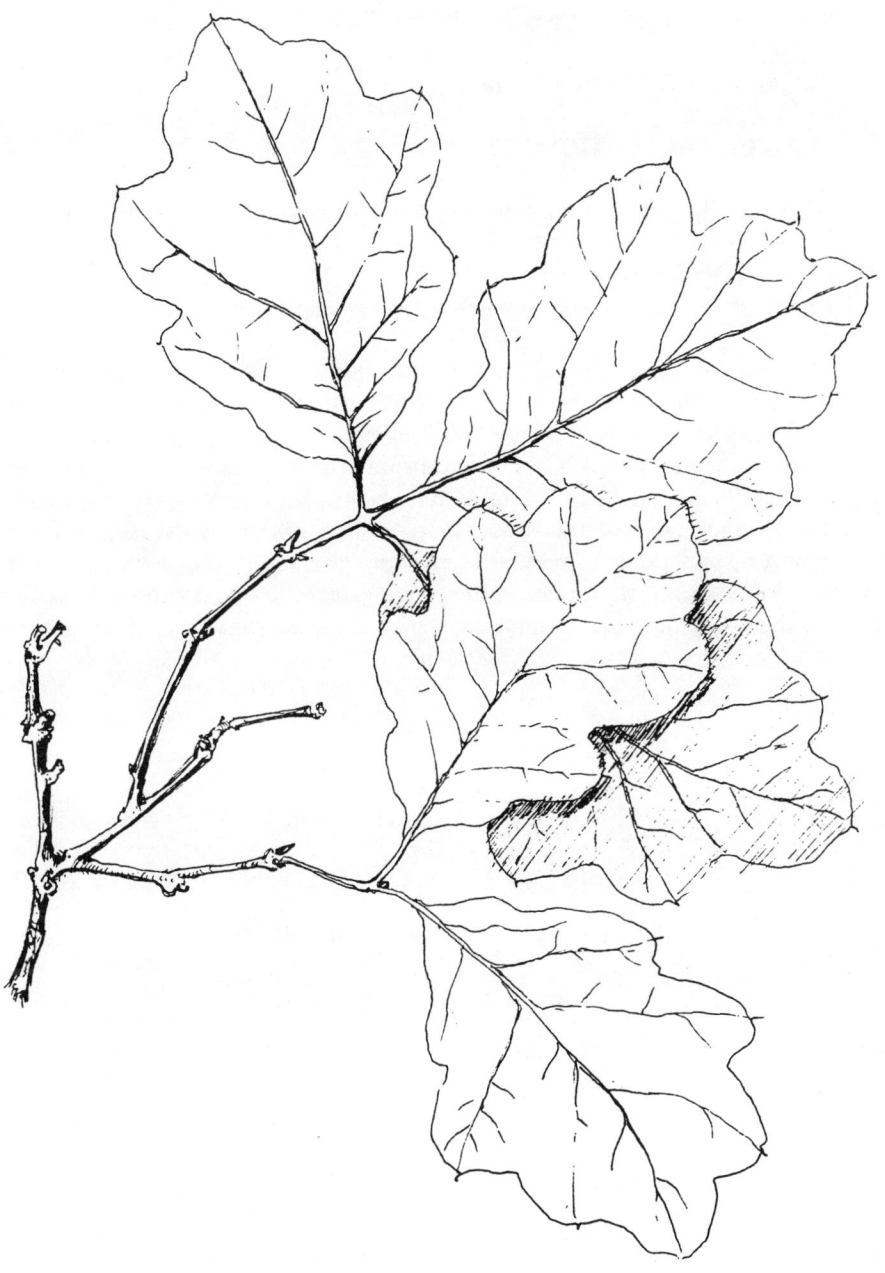

Quercus alba
White Oak

SCIENTIFIC NAME: Quercus rubra

LOCAL NAME: Red Oak Bark

LEE'S CLASSIFICATION: ST SR A

USE(S): Malaria, coughs, low or thin blood, hemorrhoids, varicose veins

ACTIVE INGREDIENTS:
Tannin; bark extract contains potash. (Felter and Lloyd: Vol. 2 1618)

Aluminum, antimony, arsenic, ash, barium, boron, bromine, cadmium, calcium, catechin, chlorine, chromium, cobalt, coniferaldehyde, copper, 2,6-dimethoxybenzoquinone, ellagic acid, europium, fluorine, gallic acid, gold, hafnium, hamamelitannin, P-hydroxybenzaldehyde, iodine, iron, lanthanum, lead, lithium, lutetium, lyoniresinol, lyoniside, magnesium, manganese, molybdenum, nickel, phosphorus, potassium, propioguaiacone, resorcin, rubidium, samarium, scandium, scopoletin, selenium, silicon, silver, sinapaldehyde, sodium, strontium, sulfur, syringaldehyde, string-aresinol, tannin, tantalum, thorium, tin, titanium, tung-sten, uranium, vanadium. (*FNF:* 148-49)

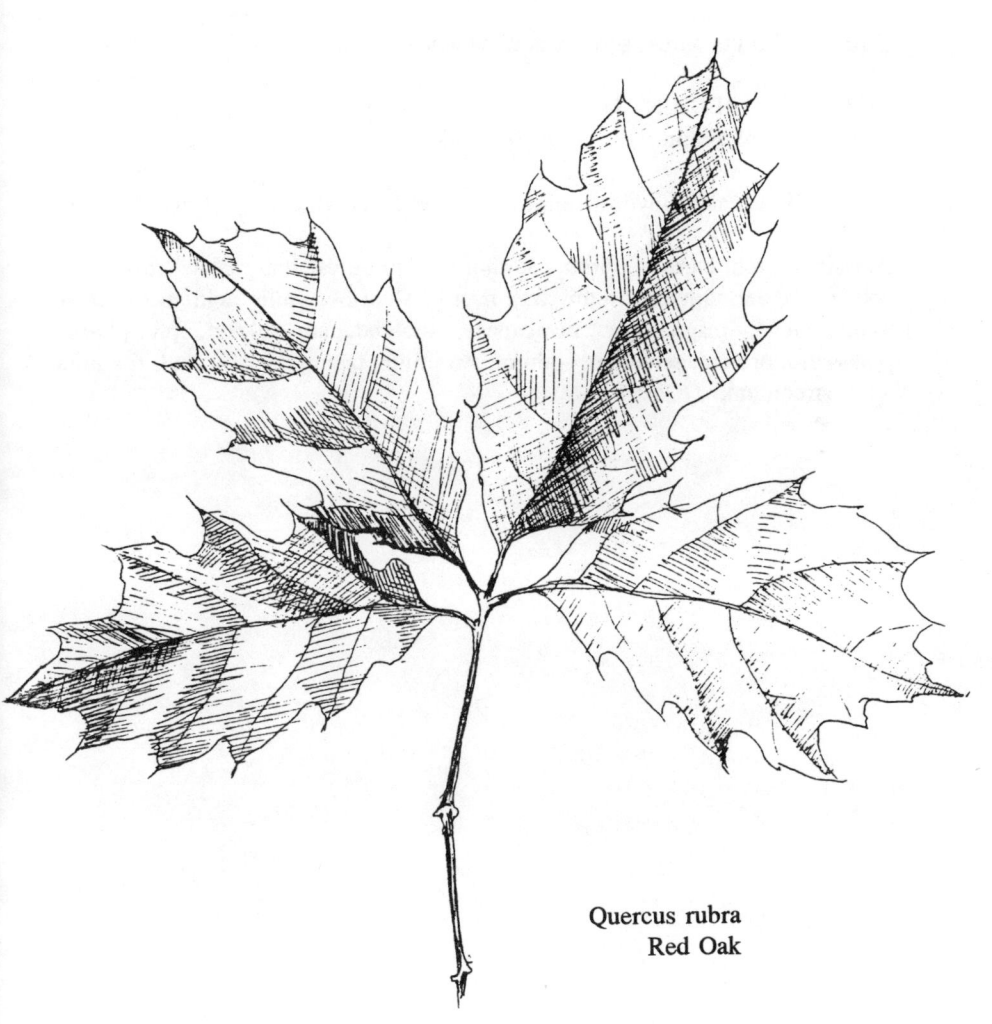

Quercus rubra
Red Oak

SCIENTIFIC NAME: Rhus glabra

LOCAL NAME: Red Sumac (Smooth Sumac)

LEE'S CLASSIFICATION: ST SR A

USE(S): Mouth sores, sore throats, wounds

ACTIVE INGREDIENTS:
Rich source of tannin. (*Wealth of Ind.*: 18)

Leaves: fisetin and dihydrofisetin, tannin, and methylgallate. (*Hagers:* 127)

Aluminum, ash, barium, boron, cadmium, calcium, calcium-malate, chromium, cobalt, copper, dihydrofisetin, fat, fisetin, fluorine, gallic acid methylester, iodine, lead, magnesium, manganese, molybdenum, nickel, phosphorus, potassium, protein, selenium, sodium, strontium, tannin, tartaric acid, titanium, zinc, zirconium. (*FNF:* 159-60)

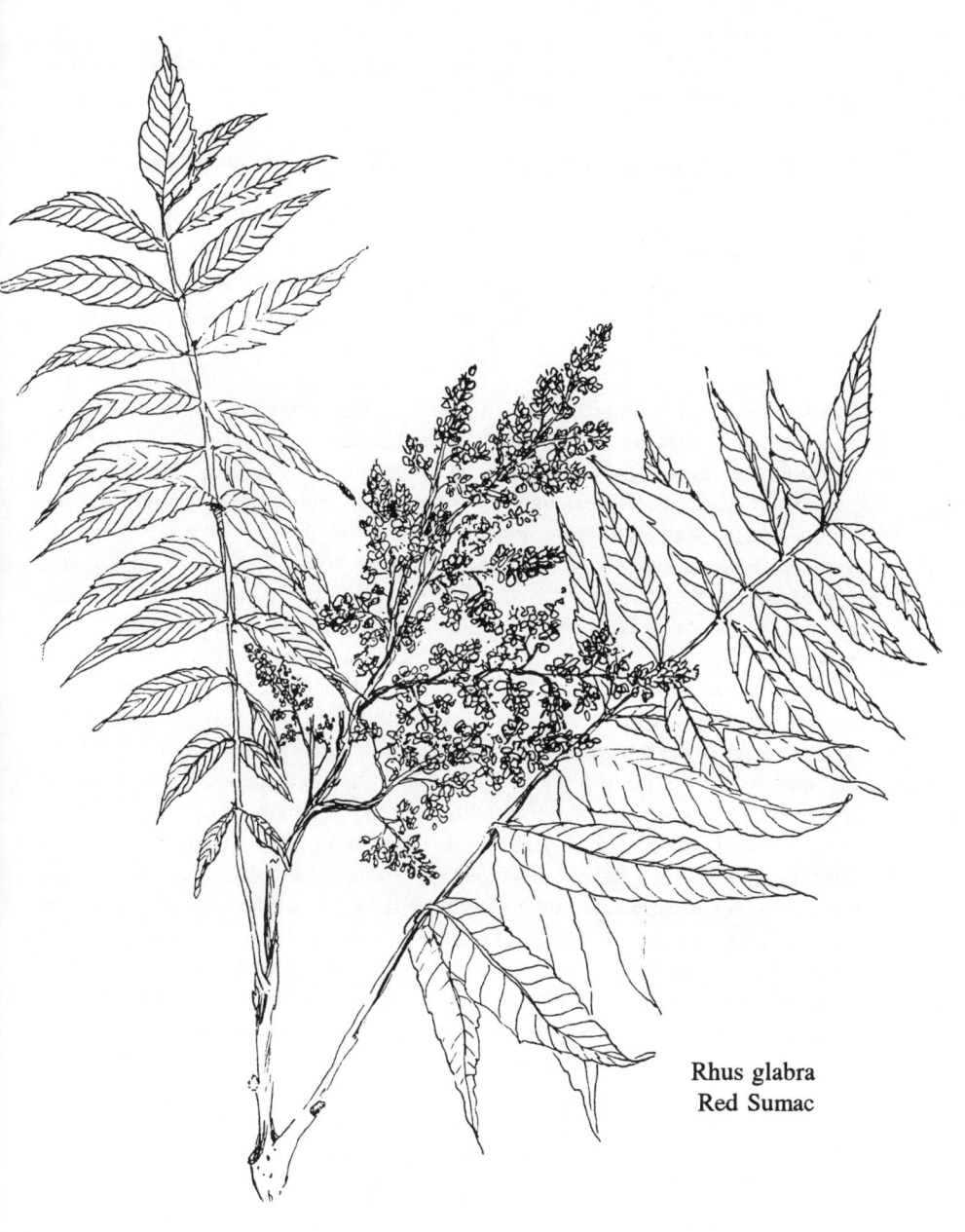

Rhus glabra
Red Sumac

SCIENTIFIC NAME: Salvia officinalis

LOCAL NAME: Sage

LEE'S CLASSIFICATION: ST SR A

USE(S): Colds, congestion, sore throats, chicken pox, menstrual cramps, headaches

ACTIVE INGREDIENTS:
Leaves: tannin, fumaric, malic, and oxalic acids, picrosalvin, saponins, pentoses; Seeds: an oil which contains oleic, linoleic, linolenic, and saturated acids. (Duke: 421)

Alpha-amyrin, beta-amyrin, alloaromadendrene, apigenin, aromadendrene, ascorbic acid, asparagine, borneol, bornyl-acetate, gamma-cadinene, delta-cadinene, calamene, calcium, camphene, camphor, 3-carene, carnosic-acid, carnosolic acid, beta-carotene, caryophyllene, beta-caryophyllene, caryophyllene-oxide, catechin, chlorogenic acid, 1,8-cineole, cirsilion, cirsimaritrin, beta-copaene, alpha-corocalene, P-coumarioc acid, P-cymene, P-cymen, dipentene-O-diphenol-lactone, EO, farnesol, fat, fumaric acid, genkwanin, germanicol, glutamine, alpha-gurjunene, trans-3-hexenal, hispidulin, alpha-humulene, iron, isocaryophyllene, labiatic acid, ledene, limonene, linalyl-acetate, linalool, linoleic acid, linolenic acid, luteolin, luteolin-7-methyl-ether, gamma-maaliene, malic acid, 6-methoxygenkwanin, 6-methoxy-genkwanin-7-methyl-ether, 6-methoxyluteolin, 6-methoxy-luteolin-7-methyl-ether, methyl-isovalerate, 2-methyl-3-methylene-5-heptane, myrcene, nepetin, niacin, nicotinic acid amide, trans-ocimene, trans-allo-ocimene, alpha-oleanolic acid, beta-oleanolic acid, oleic acid, 1-octen-3-Ol, oxalic acid, phosphorus, picrosalvin, alpha-pinene, beta-pinene, potassium, potassium-nitrate, protein, resin, riboflavin, rosmarinic acid, sabinol, sabinyl-acetate, salvigenin, salvin, salvin-methyl-ether, saponin, selina-5,11-diene, beta-sitosterol, beta-sitosterol-D-glucoside, sodium, tannin, terpinen, alpha-terpinene, gamma-terpinene, alpha-terpineol, delta-terpineol, terpineolene, thiamin, alpha-thujone, beta-thujone, (-)-thujone, thymol, N-triaco-nate, alpha-ursolic acid, beta-ursolic-acid, uvanol, viridi-floral, water, wax. (*FNF:* 181-83)

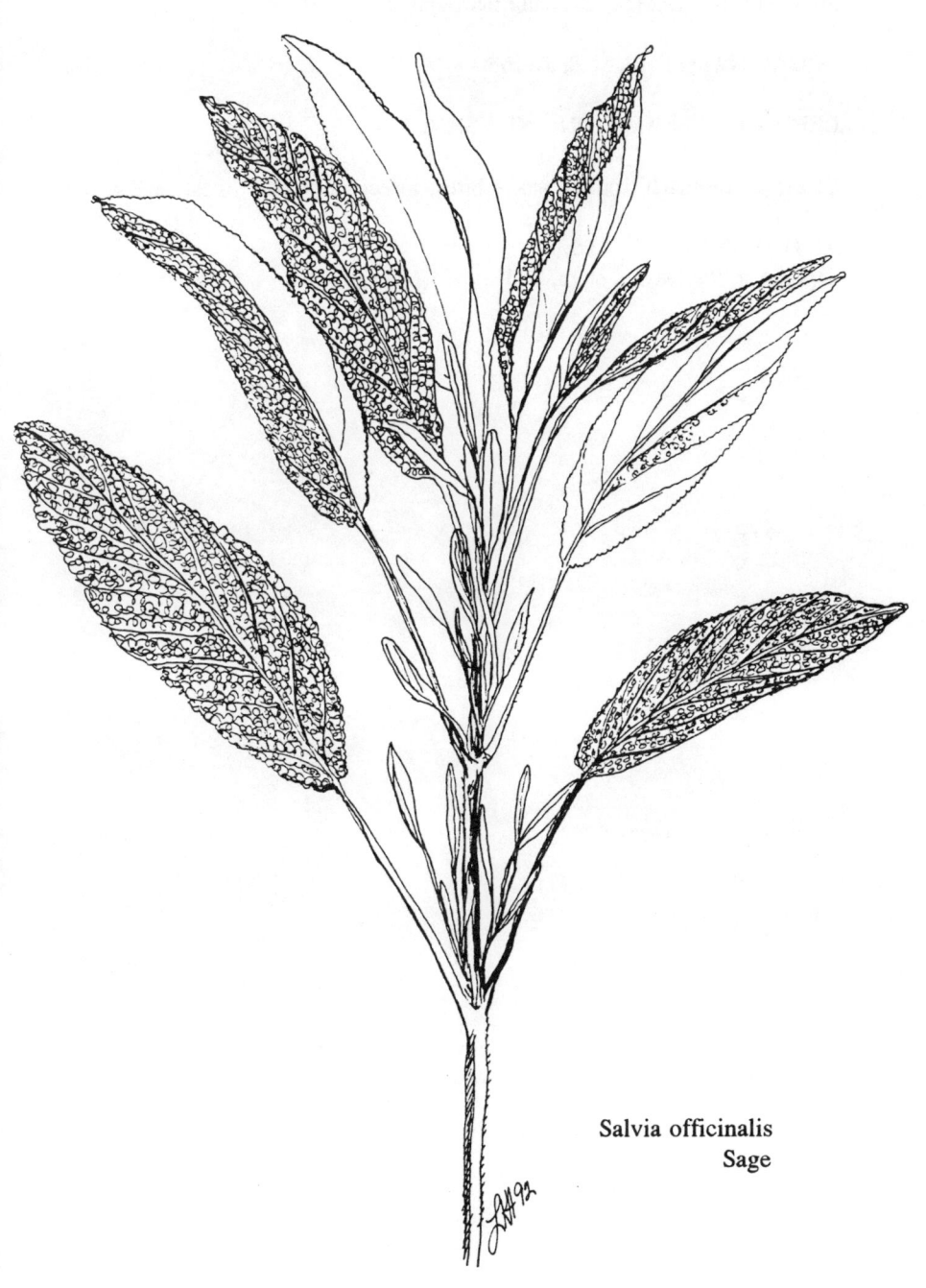

Salvia officinalis
Sage

SCIENTIFIC NAME: Sanicula marilandica

LOCAL NAME: Black Snakeroot

LEE'S CLASSIFICATION: ST VSR A

USE(S): Stomach trouble, snake bites, insect and spider bites, fevers, sores

ACTIVE INGREDIENTS:
Saponin in the leaves, stem, and root. (*Hagers:* 247)

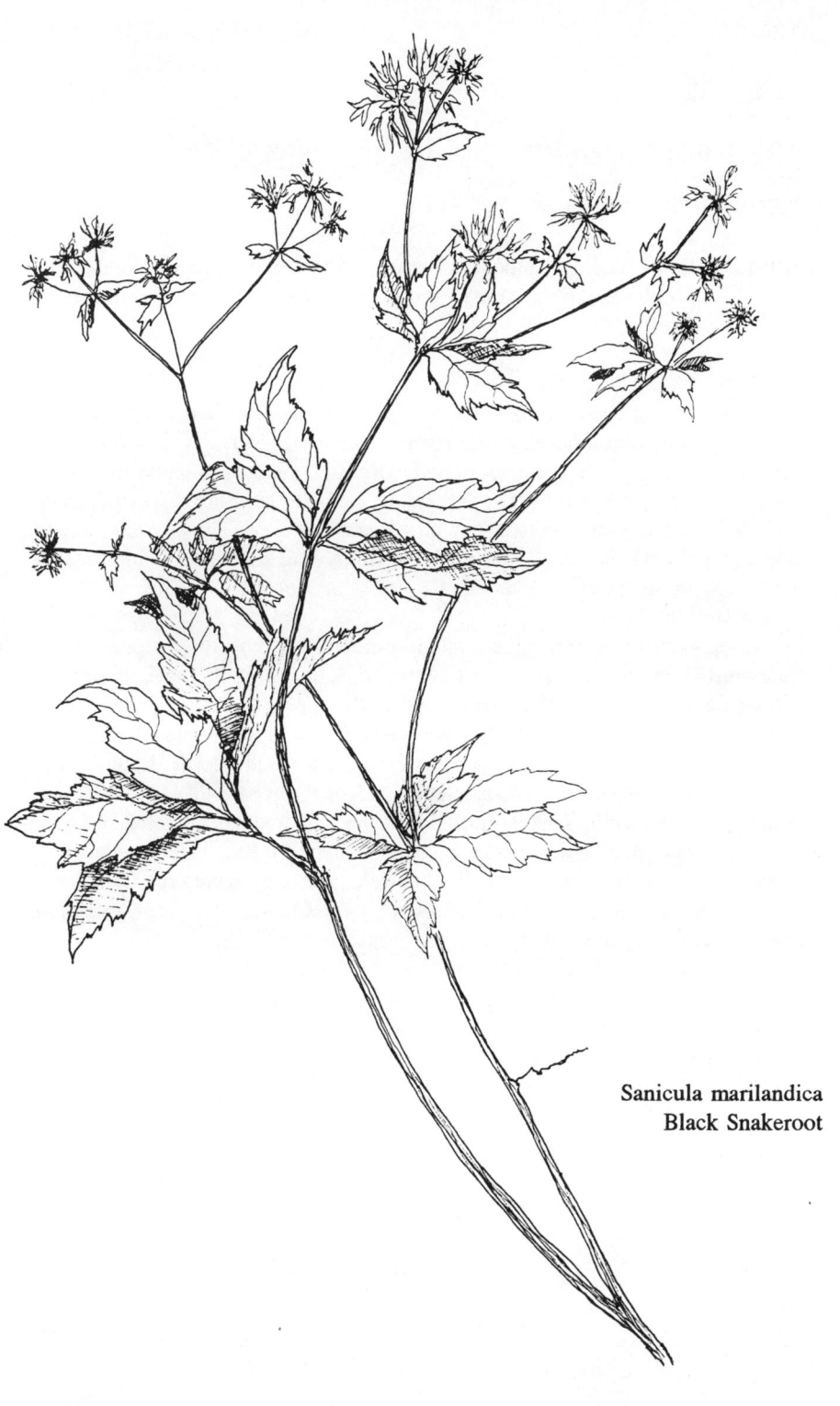

Sanicula marilandica
Black Snakeroot

SCIENTIFIC NAME: Sassafras albidium

LOCAL NAME: Sassafras

LEE'S CLASSIFICATION: MT MR A

USE(S): Bad (unclean) blood, external body sores, stomach and bowel problems, colds, kidney problems, body run down (spring tonic), swelling

ACTIVE INGREDIENTS:
Volatile oil contains safrole, some anethole, apiole, asarone, camphor, caryophyllene, coniferaldehyde copaene, elemicin, eugenol, 1-menthone, 5-methoxyeugenol, myristicin, phellandrene, pinene, piperonylacrolein sesquiterpenes, thujone. The alkaloids include boldine, cinnamolaurine, isoboldine, norboldine, norcinnamolaurine, and reticuline. Two lignins, sesamin and desmethy-oxyaschantin, are reported along with sitosterol, gum mucilage, resin, tannin, and wax. (Duke: 431)

Alkaloids, aluminum, anethole, apiole, asarone, ash, barium, boldine, boron, calcium, D-camphor, capric acid, caprylic acid, caryophyllene, chromium, cinnamolaurine, citral, cobalt, coniferaldehyde, copaene, copper, desmethyoxy-aschantin,D-2,3-dihydroxy-1-(3,4-methylendioxyphenyl)-propane,elemicin,EO, eugenol, fat, gallium, iron, iso-boldine, lauric acid, lead, linoleic acid, magnesium, manganese, L-menthone, 5-methoxyeugenol, molybdenum, mucilage, myristicin, nickel, norboldine, norcinnamolaurine, oleic acid, D-phellandrene, phellandrene, phosphorus, alpha-pinene, piperonylacrolein, potassium, protein, resin, reticuline, safrene, safrole, scandium, D-sesamin, silver, beta-sitosterol, strontium, tannin, thujone, titanium, tungsten, vanadium, zinc, zirconium. (*FNF:* 190-91)

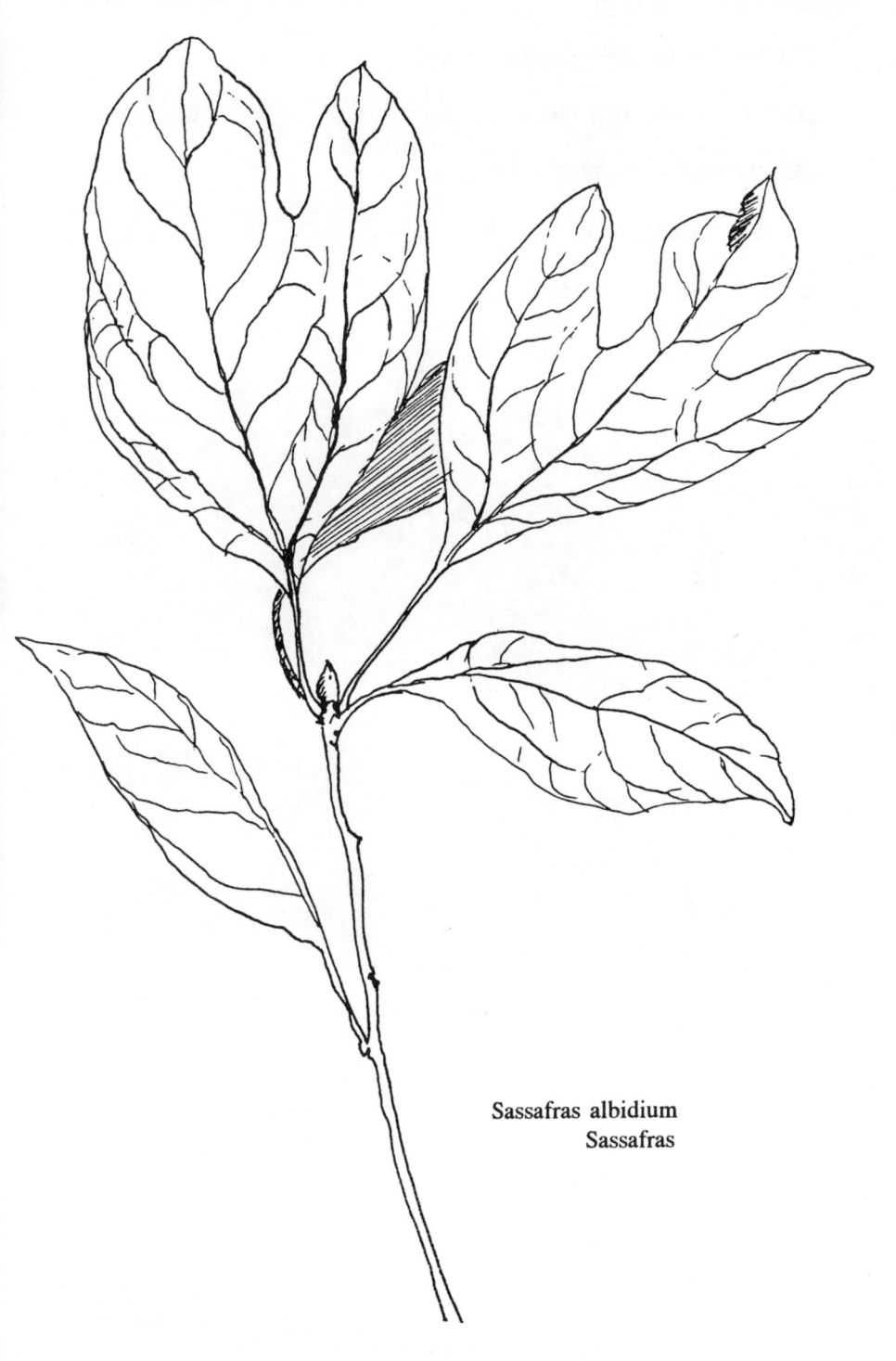

Sassafras albidium
Sassafras

SCIENTIFIC NAME: Sisyrinchium spp.

LOCAL NAME: Grip Grass

LEE'S CLASSIFICATION: ST SR A

USE(S): Constipation

ACTIVE INGREDIENTS:
No references found for this herb.

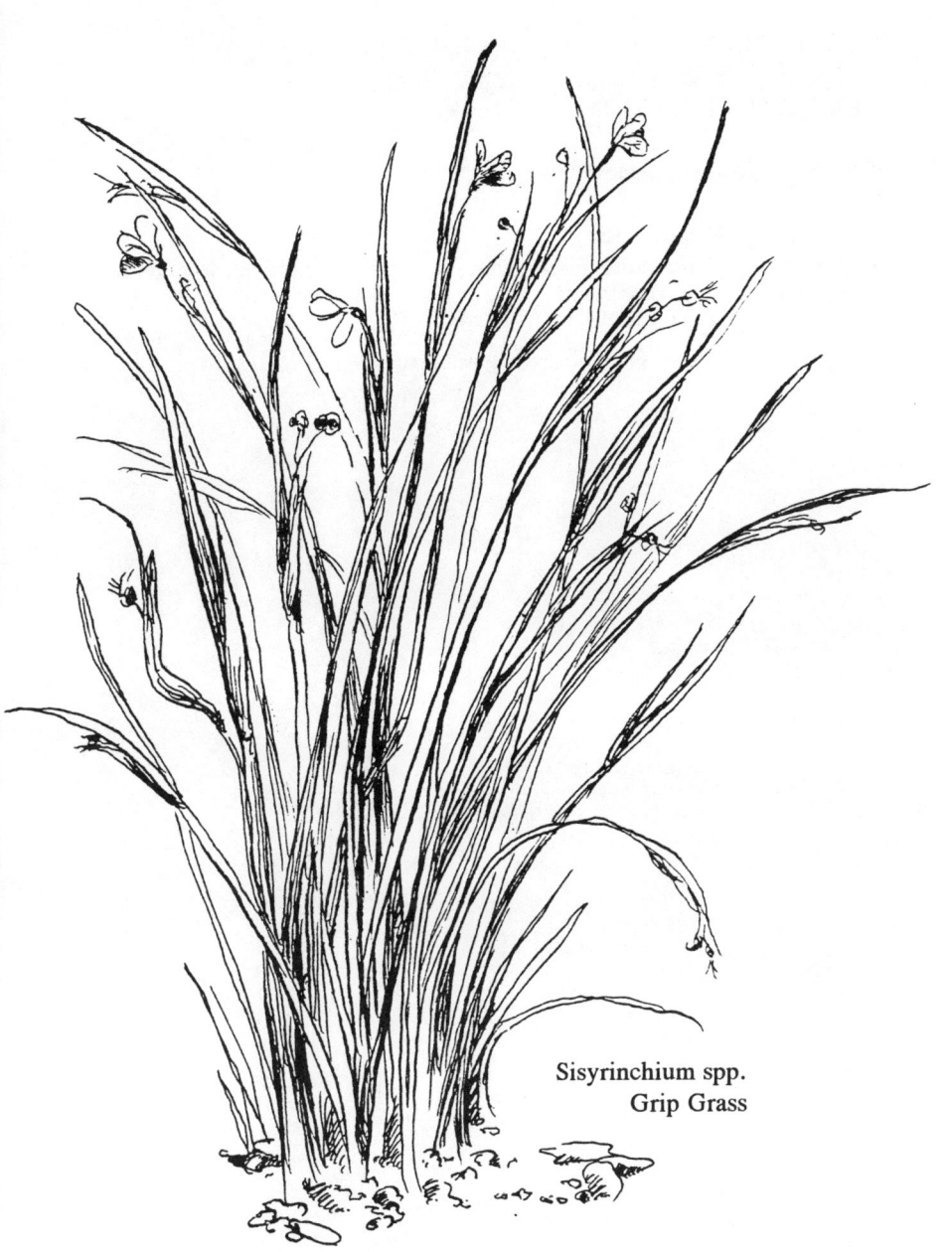

Sisyrinchium spp.
Grip Grass

SCIENTIFIC NAME: Solanum carolinense

LOCAL NAME: Dog Nettle (Horse Nettle)

LEE'S CLASSIFICATION: VST SR VA

USE(S):   Venereal disease

ACTIVE INGREDIENTS:
Leaves, berries, and roots: petroleum-ether, ether, solanidine, solnine, solanine. (Felter and Lloyd: 1800-01)

Solamargine, solasodine, solasonine, solamargine.   (*FNF:* 208)

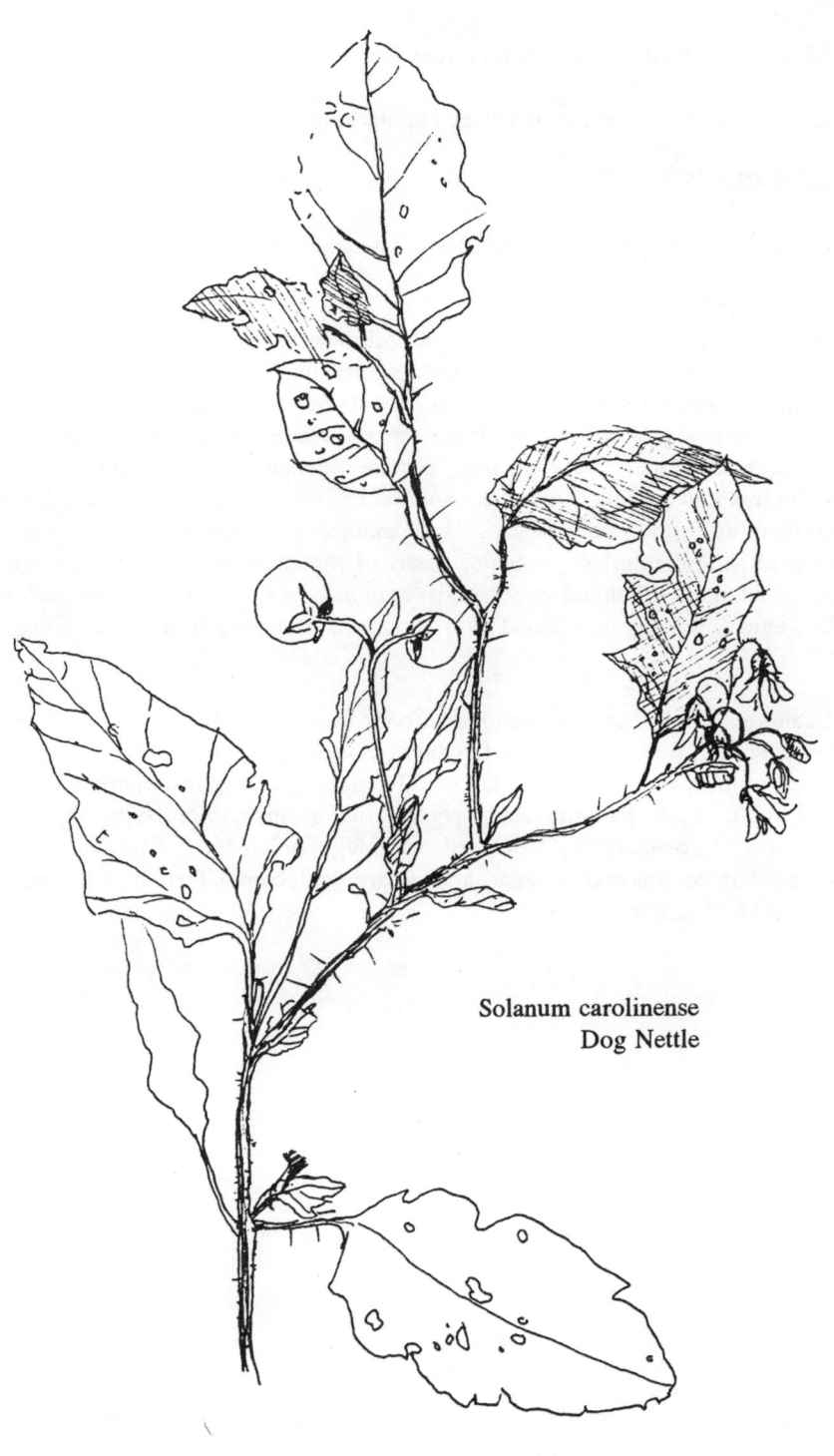

Solanum carolinense
Dog Nettle

SCIENTIFIC NAME: Solanum nigrum

LOCAL NAME: Nightshade (Black Nightshade)

LEE'S CLASSIFICATION: ___ SR A Powerful

USE(S): Poison ivy, insect bites, bee or wasp stings, rashes

ACTIVE INGREDIENTS:
Leaves: thiamine, riboflavin, niacin, ascorbic acid; Fruits: glucose, fructose, diosgenin, tigonenin; Component fatty acids: linoleic, oleic, palmitic, and stearic. Sitosterol and cholesterol also reported; Roots, shoots, and mature fruits: low in alkaloids but green fruits contain solanine which can be separated into alpha-solanine, beta-solanine, gamma-solanine, alpha-chaconine, beta-chaconine, and gamma-chaconine. Solasodine, solasonine, solamargine, beta-solamargine and alpha-beta-solansodamine, (L-rhamnosyl-D-glucosyl)-solasoidine, -solanigrine gitogenin, traces of saponins and tannins. Diploid, tetraploid, and hexaploid populations examined and significant amounts of diosgenin and solasodine found with maximum occurring in diploid. (Duke: 450)

Alkaloids, ascorbic acid, calcium, carbohydrates, beta-carotene, chaconine, cholesterol, citric acid, desgalac-totigonin, diosgenin, fat, fiber, fructose, 26-0-(beta-D-glucopyranosyl)-22-methoxy-250-5-alpha...CCO, glucose, iron, linoleic acid, oleic acid, palmitic acid, phosphorus, protein, riboflavin, saponin, sitosterol, solamargine, beta-solamargine, solanine, XI-solaninigrin, solansodamine, sola-sodine, solasonine, stearic acid, tannin, thiamin, tigo-genin, water. (*FNF:* 210)

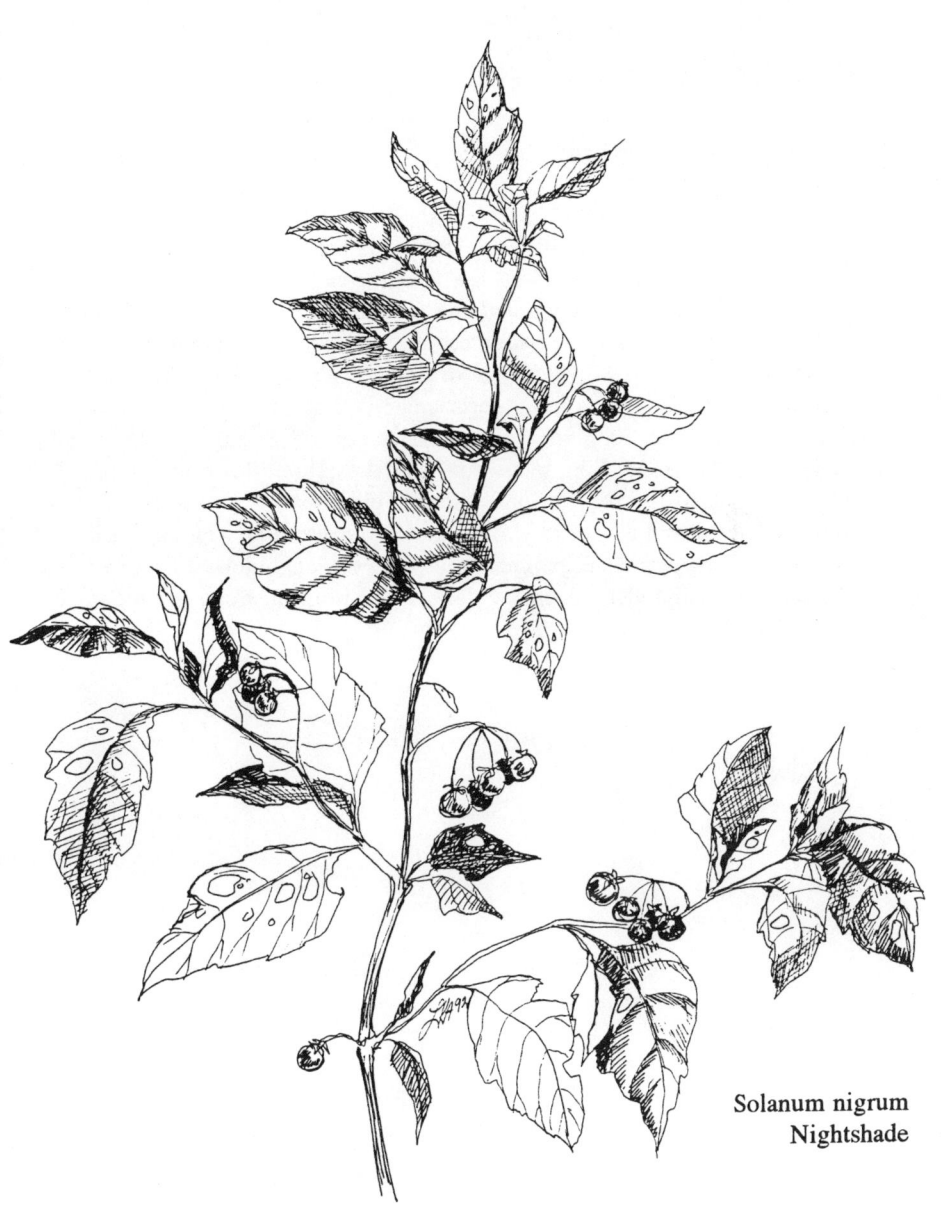

Solanum nigrum
Nightshade

SCIENTIFIC NAME: Tanacetum vulgare

LOCAL NAME: Tansy

LEE'S CLASSIFICATION: VST VSR VA

USE(S): Menstrual cramps

ACTIVE INGREDIENTS:
Arbusculin-A, artemisia-alcohol, artemisia-ketone, arte-morin, alpha-bergamotene, borneol, bornyl-acetate, gamma-cadinene, caffeic acid, alpha-campholenol, camphor, caryo-phyllene, chlorogenic acid, CIS-chrysanthenyl-acetate, trans-chrysanthenyl-acetate, 1,8-cineole, costunolide-diepoxide, crispolide, davanone, 11,13-dehydrodesacetyl-matricarin, desacetylpyretrosin, beta-elemene, EO, eupatilin, germacrene-D, 1-beta-hydroxyarbusculin-A, isochlorogenic acid, isopinocamphone, isothujone, jaceidin, jaceosidin, CIS-longipinane-2,7-dione, 1-epi-ludovicin-C, lyratrol, lyratryl-acetate, parthenolide allergenic, phyto-sterols, alpha-pinene, piperitone, reynosin, sabinene, santamarine, tanacetin allergenic, tanacetol-A, tanacetol-B, tannins, tatridine-A, tatridin-B, alpha-terpinene, gamma-terpinene, 4-thujen-2-alpha-YL-acetate, beta-thujone, beta-thujyl-alcohol, umbellulone, viburnitol, vulgarone-A, vulgarone-B.
(*FNF:* 228-29)

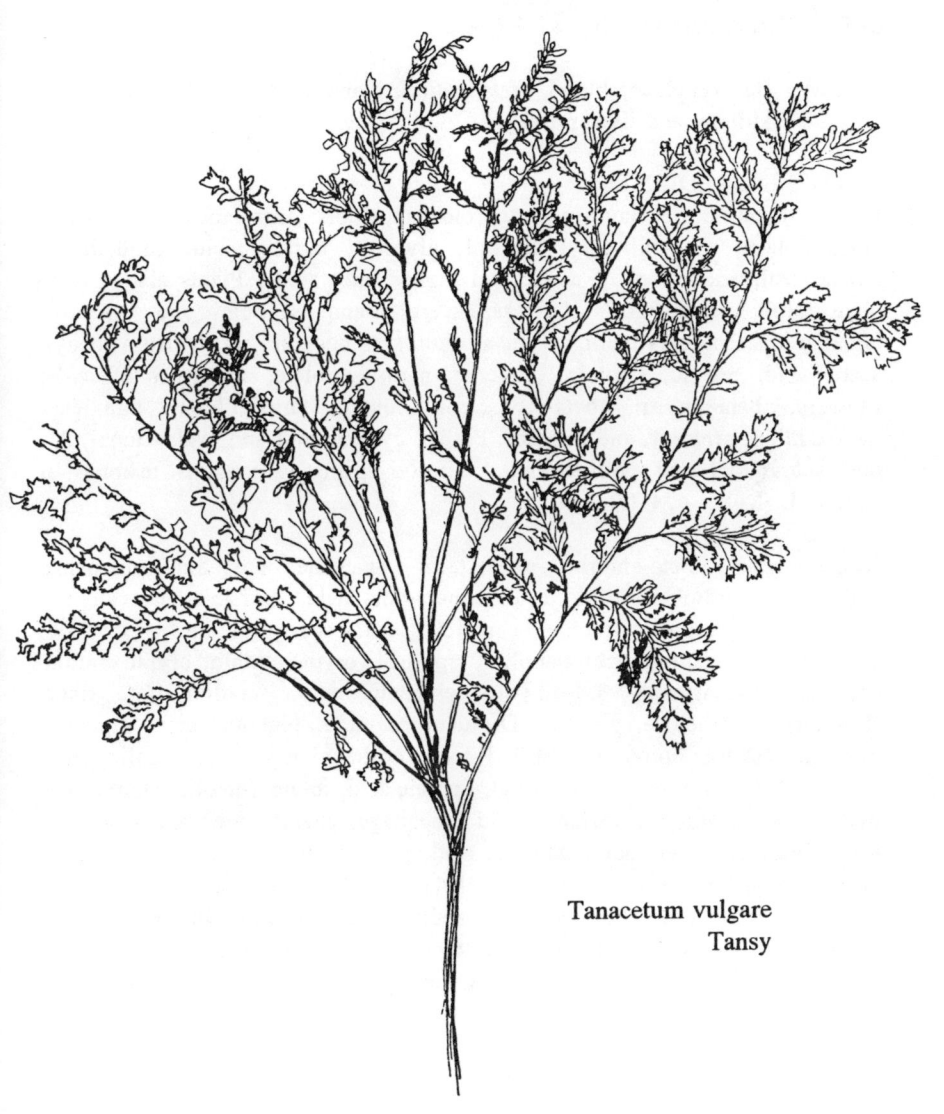

Tanacetum vulgare
Tansy

SCIENTIFIC NAME: Taraxacum officinale

LOCAL NAME: Dandelion

LEE'S CLASSIFICATION: ST SR A

USE(S): Bad (unclean) blood, constipation, diabetes, fevers, urinary tract, kidney, and liver problems

ACTIVE INGREDIENTS:
Leaves: thiamine, riboflavin, and ascorbic acid; Roots: taraxacine, inulin, glutin, gum, potash; Latex: ceryl alcohol, glycerin, tartaric acid, caoutchouc, taraxasterol, and esters of acetic and higher fatty acids; Plants also contain phytosterols taraxasterol, homotaraxsterol, and saponin and rosterol, homoandrosterol, cluytianol, cerylic alcohol, arabinose and beta hydroxyphenyl-acetic acid, cerotic, linoleic, linolenic, melissic, oleic, and palmitic acids; Flowers: beta-amyrin, beta-sistosterol, lutein, taraxanthine, taraxiene, flavoxanthin, arnidiol, and faradiol; Pollen: cycloartenol and cycloartanol, 31-nor-cycloartanol and pollinastanol. In the spring it contains mannite or mannitol. (Duke: 474-77)

Alpha-amylase, beta-amyrin, androsterol, aneurine, apigenin-7-glucoside, arabinose, arnidiol, ascorbic acid, asparaginic acid, caffeic acid, calcium, caoutchouc, carbohydrates, cerotic acid, certyl-alcohol, choline, chrysanthemumxanthin, cluytianol, coumestrol, cryptoxanthin, cryptoxanthin-epoxide, cycloartanol, 3,4-dihydroxycinnamic acid, faradiol, fat, fiber, flavoxanthin, fructose, glucose, D-glucuronic acid, glutamic acid, glycerol, homoandrosterol, homotraxasterol, P-hydroxyphenyl acetic acid, inulin, iron, lactucerol, lecithin, levulin, levulose, linoleic acid, lutein, luteolin-7-glucoside, magnesium, mannitol, melissic acid, mucilage, niacin, nicotinic acid, 31-norcycloartenol, oleic acid, palmitic acid, pectins, phlobaphene, phosphorus, pollinastanol, potassium, protein, pseudotaraxasterol, resin, riboflavin, saccharose, saponin, beta-sitosterol, sodium, stigmasterol, sucrose, tannin, taraxacerine, taraxacine, taraxanthin, taraxasterol, taraxerol, taraxol, tartaric acid, thiamin, tyrosinase, violaxanthin, xathophyll, water. (*FNF:* 230-32)

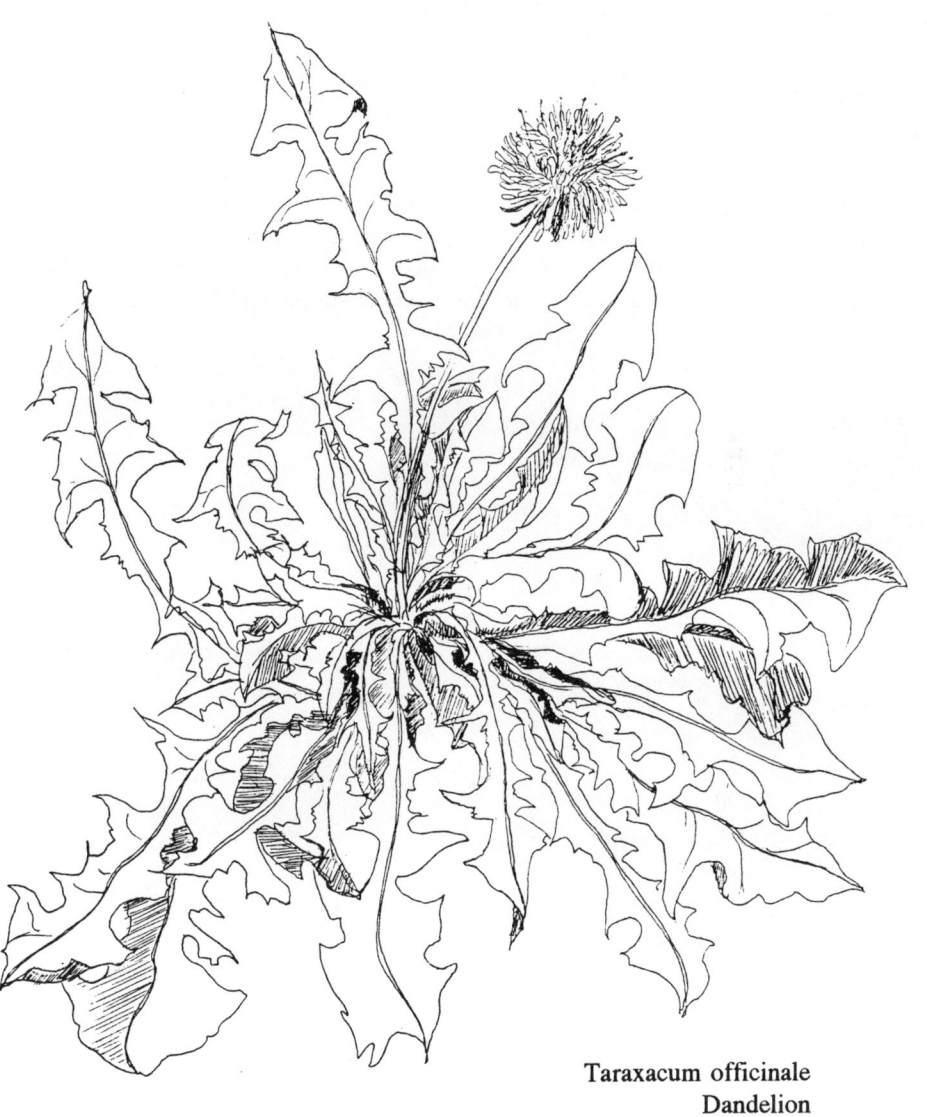

Taraxacum officinale
Dandelion

SCIENTIFIC NAME: Trifolium pratense

LOCAL NAME: Red Clover

LEE'S CLASSIFICATION: MT MR MA

USE(S): Arthritis, cancer, liver troubles

ACTIVE INGREDIENTS:
Seeds: trypsin inhibitors and chymotrypsin; Plants: isoflavones formononetin, biochanin A, daidzein and genistein; Flowers: salicylic acid, p-coumaric acid, isor-hammetin, glucosides including phytosterol glucoside tri-folianol, trifolin, trifolitin, rhammose, isotrifolin, pratol, pratensol, genestein, coumestrol, trans- and cis-cloramide, phaseolic acid, and pterocarpan phytoalexins. (Duke: 489)

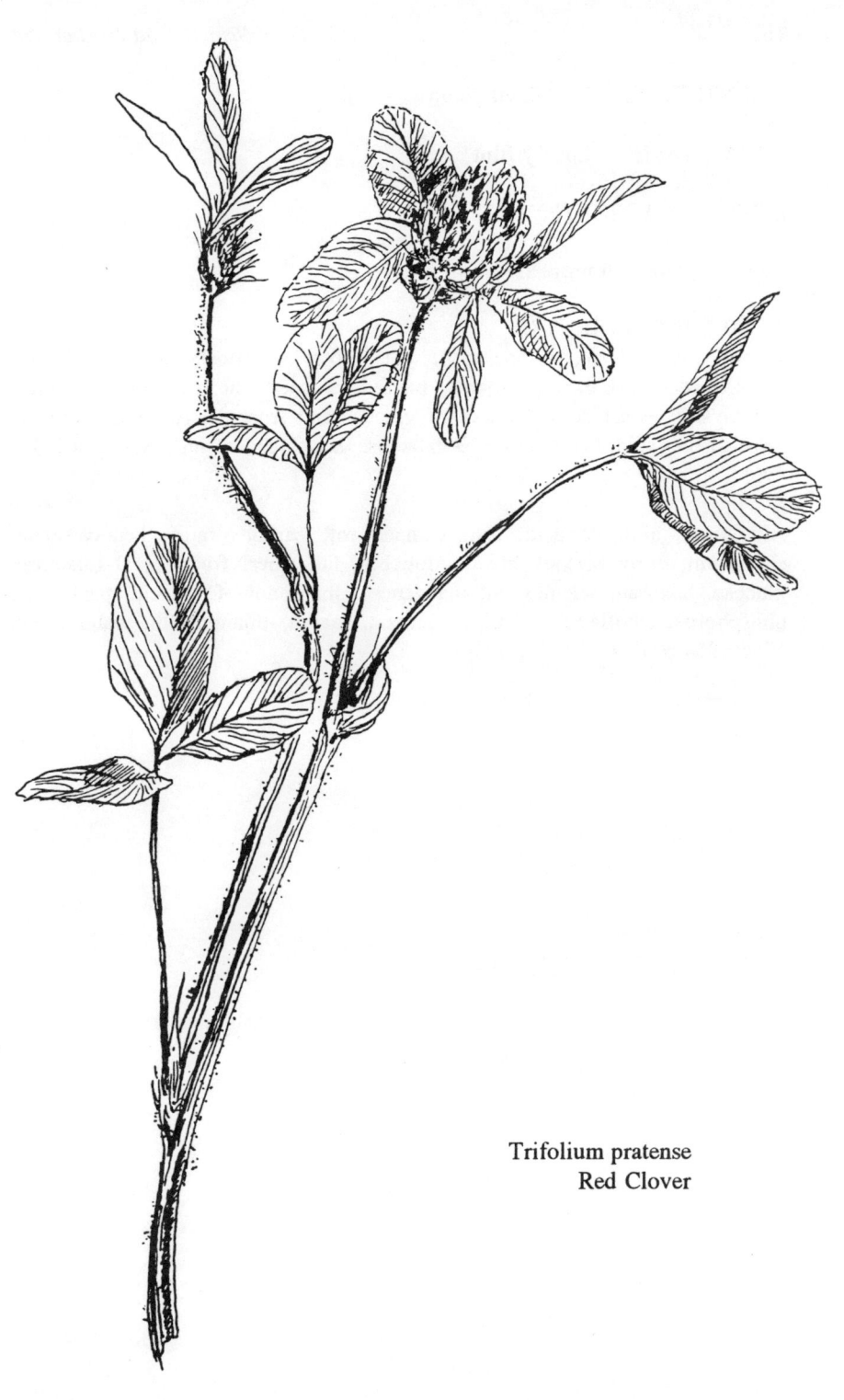

Trifolium pratense
Red Clover

SCIENTIFIC NAME: Ulmus rubra

LOCAL NAME: Slippery Elm

LEE'S CLASSIFICATION: MT SR VA

USE(S):   Stomach problems

ACTIVE INGREDIENTS:
Wood: cholesterol, campesterol, beta-sitosterol, citosta-dienol, dolichol, sesquiterpenes; Bark: pentoses, methyl-pentoses, hexoses (which after hydrolysis), galactose and traces of glucose and fructose, two polyuronides, galac-turonic acid, L-rhamnose, D-galactose, mucilage, calcium oxalate. (Duke: 496)

Aluminum, ascorbic acid, ash, campesterol, carbohydrates, beta-carotene, chromium, citrostadienol, cobalt, dolichol, fat, fiber, fructose, D-galactose, glucose, hexosan, magnesium, manganese, mansonone-C, niacin, pentosans, phosphorus, riboflavin, selenium, silicon, tannin, thiamin, tin, water, zinc. (*FNF:* 254-55)

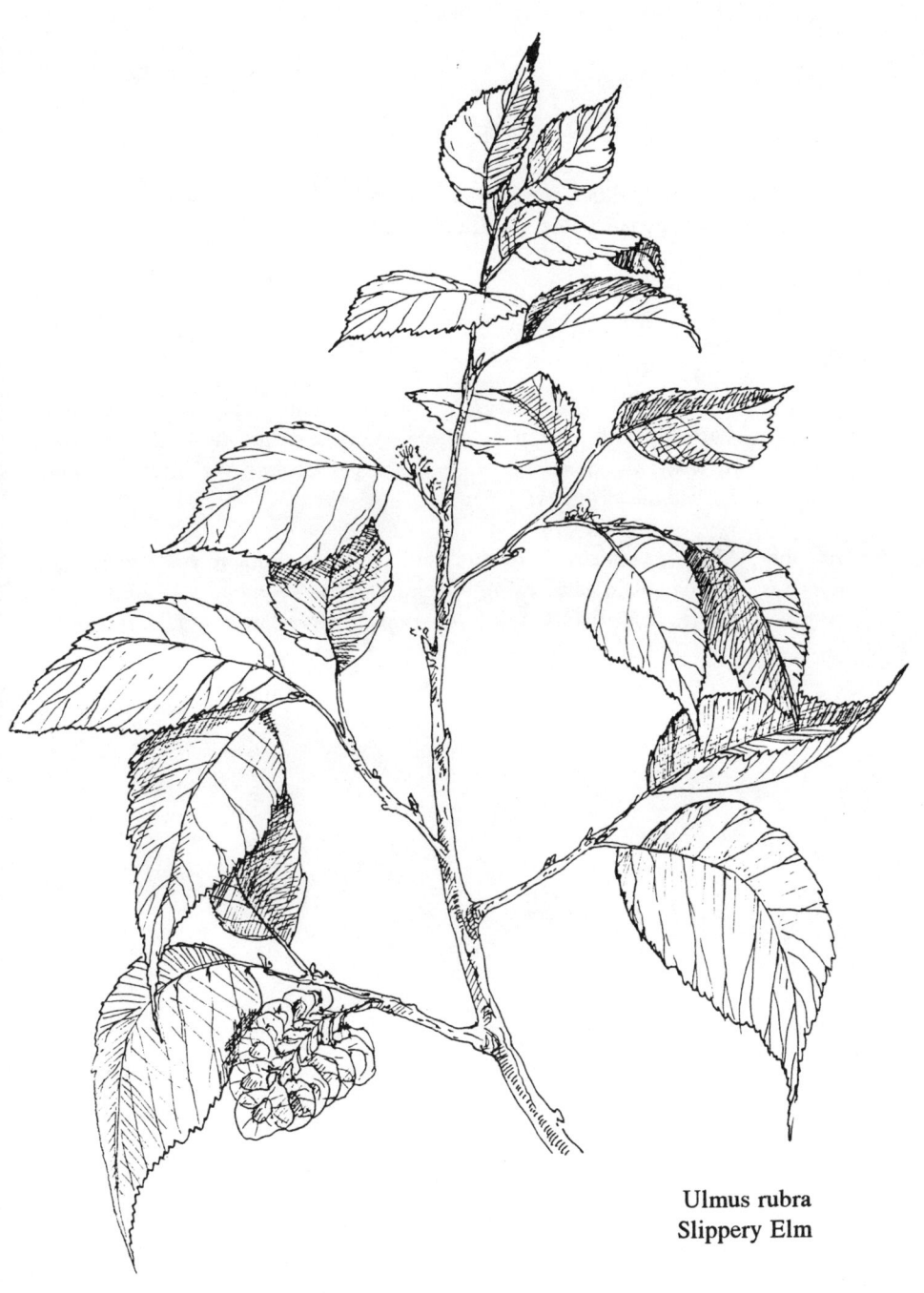

Ulmus rubra
Slippery Elm

SCIENTIFIC NAME: Verbascum thapsus

LOCAL NAME: Mullein

LEE'S CLASSIFICATION: ST SR A

USE(S): Coughs, asthma, congestion, sore throat, colds, stomach trouble, bed sores, hemorrhoids, swelling, wounds, warts

ACTIVE INGREDIENTS:
Leaves: rotenone, coumarin, and several saponins; Flowers: crocetin. (*Wealth of Ind.*: 444-45)

Leaves: saponin, mucilage, bitterings, rotenone, and resin; Seeds: saponin, mucilage, fatty oil with glycerides of oleic acid and linoleic acid; Blossom: thapsic acid; Root: verba-cose, coumarin, and phytosterin, verbasterol; Other: catapol and aucubin. (*Hagers:* 420)

Aucubin, catapol, coumarin, crocetin, fat, heptaose, linoleic acid, mucilage, nonaose, octaose, oleic acid, palmitic acid, protein, rotenone, saponins, beta-sitosterol, stearic acid, thapsic acid, verbascose, verbasterol. (*FNF:* 263-64)

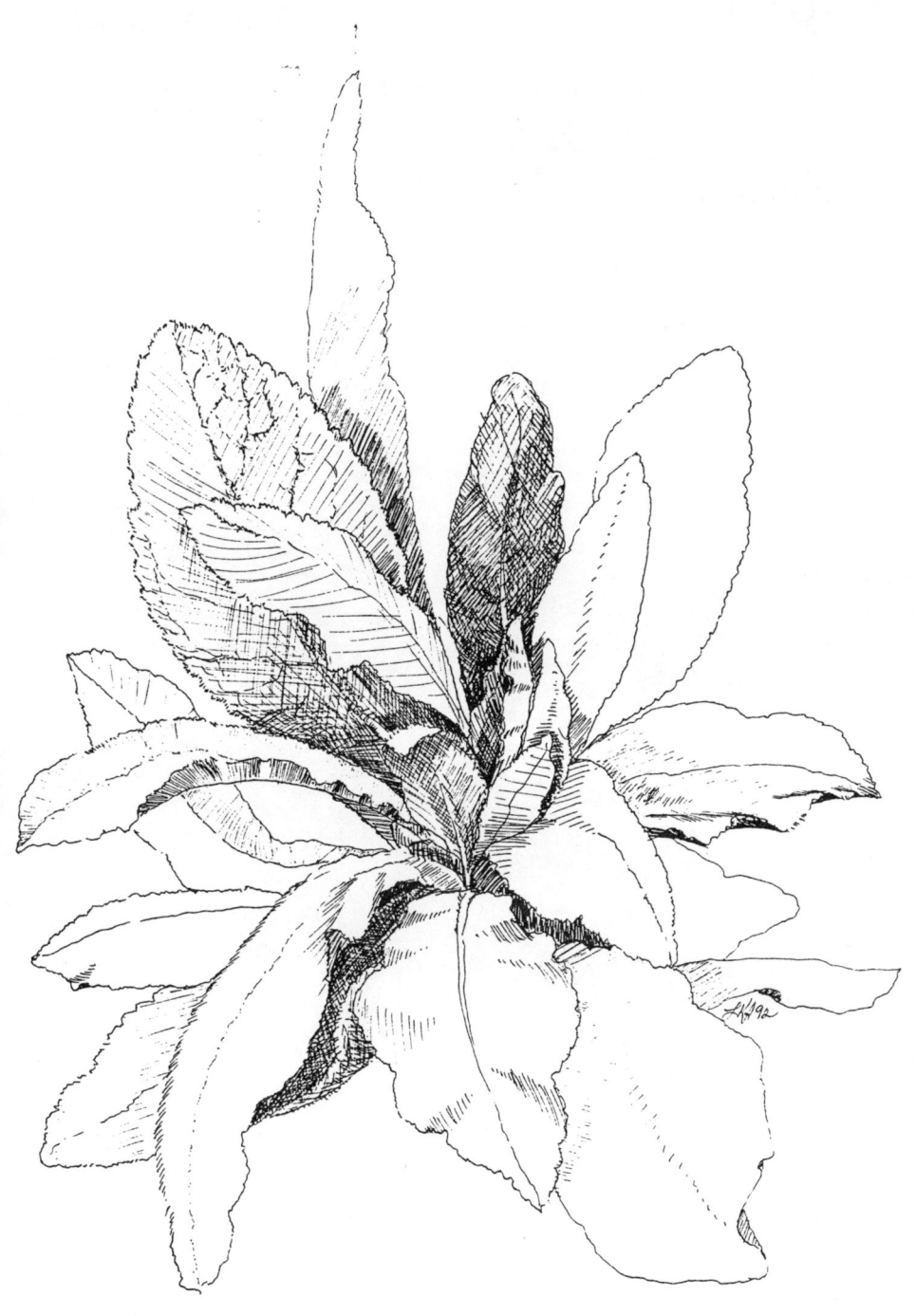

Verbascum thapsus
Mullein

SCIENTIFIC NAME: Zea mays (stigmata)

LOCAL NAME: Corn silk

LEE'S CLASSIFICATION: MT SR A

USE(S): Bedwetting, mumps

ACTIVE INGREDIENTS:
Menthol, thymol, carvacrol, alpha-terpineol, betaine, beta-sitosterol. (*Hagers:* 552)

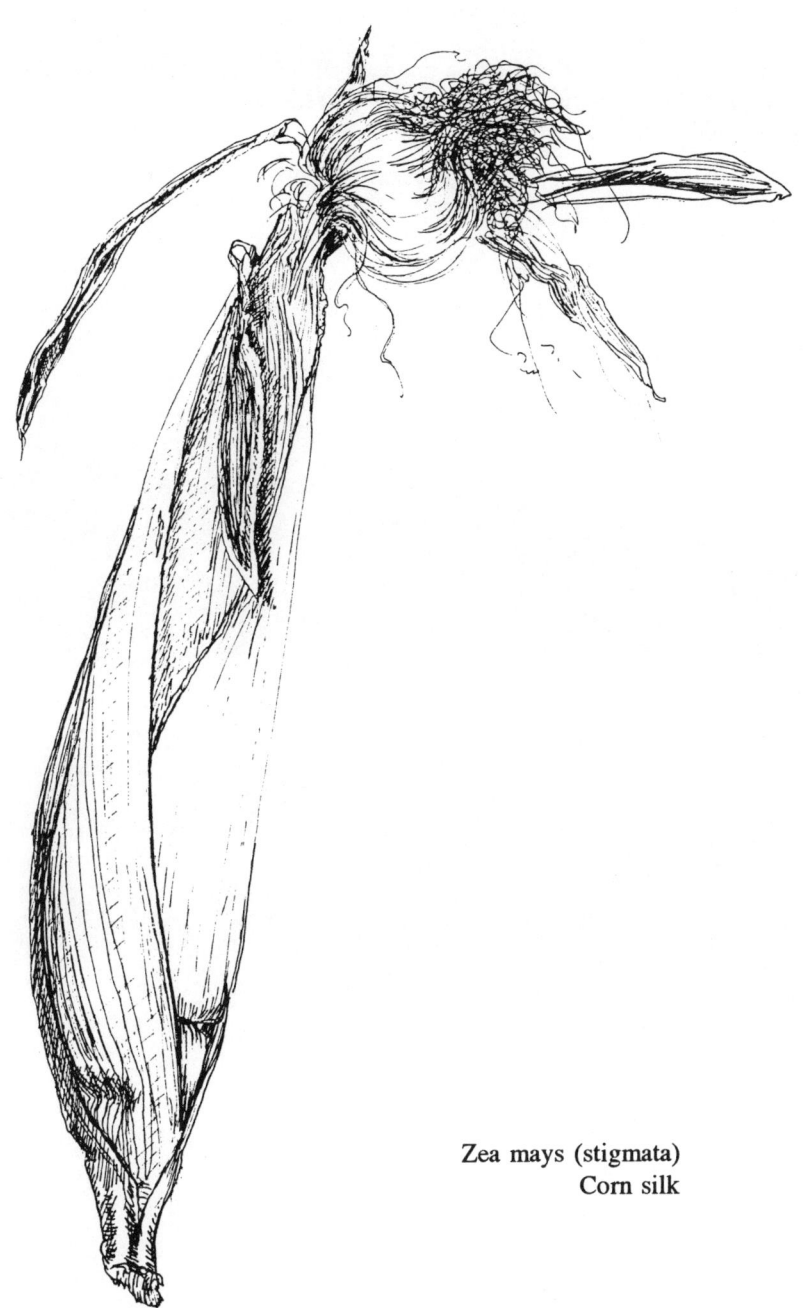
Zea mays (stigmata)
Corn silk

NOTE

1. Mr. Michael Wachholz, a graduate student in the German Department at Howard University, made the translations of the German passages in *Hager's Handbook*.

Appendix

Biologicals

COBWEBS
Cobwebs are used to stop the bleeding of cuts.
Apply the cobweb to the cut to stop the bleeding.

DIRT DAUBER
Dirt dauber nests are used for sprains, bee and wasp stings, and swellings.
Mix the nest with vinegar, and apply as a poultice on a sprain or stung area and let it dry. Apply more later if needed.

EAR WAX
Used for fever blisters.
Apply the ear wax directly on the blister.

EGG SHELL LINING
Used for boils.
Put the thin white lining of an egg shell on the boil to draw it to a head.

HEN HOUSE DROPPINGS
Used for colic and prostate gland problems.
Make a tea using hen droppings. One cup of water and one tablespoon of droppings. Take one cup two to three times a day.

HOG HOOF
Used for pneumonia, whooping cough, and coughs.
Boil the hooves and soak them in whiskey. Take one tablespoon three times a day.

HOG JAW MARROW
Used for mumps.
Split the jawbone and get out the marrow. Apply the marrow to the area of the swelling in an upward motion. Apply one to two times a day.

SHEEP DUNG
Used for shingles.
Boil one cup of sheep dung in one quart of water. Take three fourths cup two to three times a day.

SOOT
Used for cuts.
Apply the soot to the cut to stop the bleeding. Put the soot on first and then apply cobwebs.

References

Anderson, Jean. *Piedmont Plantation: The Bennehan-Camerson Family and Lands in North Carolina.* Durham, N.C.: The Historic Preservation Society of Durham, 1985.

Ackernecht, Erwin H. "Primitive Medicine and Culture Pattern." *Bulletin of Historical Medicine.*, 12, 1942: 545-574.

Ackernecht, Erwin H. *Medicine and Thenology: Selected Essays.* Baltimore: Johns Hopkins University Press, 1971.

Angier, Bradford. *Field Guide to Medicinal Wild Plants.* Harrisburg, Penn.: Stackpole Books, 1978.

Ayensu, Edward S. *Medicinal Plants of West Africa.* Mich.: Reference Publications, 1978.

Bannerman, Robert, John Burton, and Ch'en Wen-Chieh, eds. *Traditional Medicine and Health Care Coverage.* Geneva: World Health Organization (WHO), 1983.

Berlin, Ira. "Time, Space, and the Evolution of Afro-American Society on British Mainland North America." *American Historical Review,* 85(1): 44-78, 1980.

Bhagrat, Singh. *A Short History of Aryan Medicine.* Gondal, India: Shree Bhagavat Jee Electric Printing Press, 1927.

Blaustein, Richard. "Traditional Healing Today: Moving Beyond Stereotypes," in Holly Mathews et. al, eds., *Traditional Medicine in the South Today.* Durham, N.C.: Duke University Press, 32-40, 1992.

Bontemps, Arna. *Great Slave Narratives.* Boston: Beacon Press, 1969.

Braun, Emma. L. *Deciduous Forests of Eastern North America.* New York: Hafner Publishing. Company, 1964.

Cohen, Lucy, and Tim Ready, eds., *Field Training in Applied Anthropology.* Vol. 3. Washington, D.C.: Department of Anthropology, Catholic University of America Press, 1984.

Collins, Alice, and Diane Pancoast. Natural Helping Networks, National Association of Social Workers. Washington, D.C., 1976.

Croom, E. "Herbal Medicine among the Lumbee Indians," in H. Mathews et al., eds., *Traditional Medicine in the South Today*. Durham: Duke University Press, 137-69, 1992.

Daniel, Pete. *Breaking the Land*. Chicago: University of Illinois Press, 1985.

de Albuquerque, Klaus. "Non-Institutional Medicine on the Sea Islands," in Melba Varner and Amy McCandless, eds., *Proceedings of a Symposium on Culture and Health Implications for Health Policy in Rural South Carolina*. Charleston, S.C.: College of Charleston, Center for Metropolitan Affairs and Public Policy, 33-78, 1979.

Deas-Moore, V. "Medical Adaptations of a Culture Relocated from Africa to the Sea Islands of South Carolina." *The World and I*, 2(1): 474-85, 1987.

Duffy, John. "A Note on Ante-Bellum Southern Nationalism and Medical Practices." *The Journal of Southern History*, 34: 268-76, 1968.

Duke, James. *C.R.C. Handbook of Medicinal Herbs*. Boca Raton, Fla.: CRC Press, 1985.

Duke, James. *Father Nature's Farmacy*, computer database, 1990.

Duke, James. *Handbook of Phytochemical Constituents of GRAS Herbs and Other Economic Plants*. Boca Raton, Fla.: CRC Press, 1992.

Duke, James. *Handbook of Biologically Active Phytochemicals and Their Activities*. Boca Raton, Fla.: CRC Press, 1992.

Durkheim, Emile. *Education and Sociology*. Translated and with an Introduction by Sherwood D. Fox. Glencoe, Illinois: Free Press, 1956.

Fabrega, Horacio. "Medical Anthroplogy," in Bernard Siegal, ed., *Biennial Review of Anthropology*. Stanford: Stanford University Press, 167-229, 1971(a).

Fabrega, Horacio. "Some Features of Zinacatecan Medical Knowledge." *Ethnology*, 10:25-43, 1971(b).

Felter, Harvey, and John Lloyd. *King's American Dispensatory*. Vols. 1 and 2, Portland, Oregon: Eclectic Medical Publications, 1983.

Filliozat, Jean. *The Classical Doctrine of Indian Medicine: Its Origins and Its Greek Parallels*, translated from the French by Dev. Raj Chanana. Delhi: Menshiram Manoharlal, 1946.

Foster, George. "Relationship between Spanish and Spanish-American Folk Medicine." *Journal of American Folklore*, 201-17, 1966.

Foster, George. "Disease Etiologies in Northwestern Medical Systems." *American Anthropologist.*, 78:771-82, 1976.

Garland, Sarah. *The Complete Book of Herbs and Spices*. New York: Viking Press, 1979.

Glick, Leonard. "Medicine as an Ethnographic Category: The Gimi at the New Guinea Highlands." *Ethnology*, 6:31-56, 1967.

References

Gordon, B. L. *Medicine through Antiquity.* Philadelphia: F. A. Davis Co., 1967.

Grieve, Maud. *A Modern Herbal.* New York: Hafner Press, 1974.

Grime, William. *Ethno-Botany of the Black Americans.* Mich.: Reference Publishing, 1976.

Gulick, John. *Cherokees at the Crossroads.* Chaptel Hill: Institute for Research in Social Science, University of North Carolina, 1960.

Hall, Arthur, and Peter Bourne. "Indigenous Therapists in a Southern Black Urban Community." *Archives of General Psychiatry,* 28: 137-42, 1973.

Hamel, Paul, and Mary Chiltoskey. *Cherokee Plants and Their Uses: A 400 Year History.* Sylvia, N.C.: Herald Publishing. Company, 1975.

Hand, Wayland. *American Folk Medicine.* Berkeley: University of California Press, 1976.

Hand, Wayland. *Magical Medicine: The Folkloric Component of Medicine in the Folk Belief, Custom, and Ritual of the Peoples of Europe and America.* Berkeley: University of California Press, 1980.

Hand, Wayland, Ana Caseta, and Sondra Thiederman, eds. *Popular Beliefs and Superstitions: A Compendium of American Folklore.* Vols. 1 and 2. From the Ohio Collection of Newbell Niles Puckett. Boston, Mass.: G. K. Holland Co., 1981.

Haufman, M. A. "Folk Health and Illness Beliefs." *Nurse Practitioner,* 4(4):23-34, 1979.

Haywood, Charles. *A Bibliography of North American Folklore and Folksong.* New York: Greenberg, 1951.

Henderson, George, and Martha Primeaux, eds., *Transcultural Health Care.* London: Addison-Wesley, 1981.

Holloway, Irene. "Hot and Cold in Mexican Folk Medicine," Department of Anthropology, University of Maryland, 1980.

Hughes, Charles. "Medical Care: Ethnomedicine," in D. Silla, ed., *International Encyclopedia of the Social Sciences.* New York: The Free Press, 1968.

Hutchinson, John, and John Dalziel. *The Useful Plants of West Tropical Africa.* London: The Crown Agents for the Colonies, 1937.

Hyatt, Harry. *Memoirs of the Alma Egan Hyatt Foundation: Hoodoo, Conjuration, Witchcraft, Rootwork.* 5 Vols. Cambridge, Mass.: Western Publishing Company, 1970-78.

Ingham, John. "On Mexican Folk Medicine." *American Anthropologist,* 72:76-87, 1970.

Jackson, Bruce. "The Other Kind of Doctor: Conjure and Magic in Black American Folk Medicine," in Wayland Hand, ed., *American Folk Medicine: A Symposium.* Berkeley: University of California Press, 259-71, 1976.

Jenkins, Abraham. "An Insider's History of the Sea Islands and Efforts to Bring Health Care to the Islanders," in Melba Varner and Amy McCandless, eds., *Proceedings of A Symposium on Culture and Health: Implications for Health Policy in Rural South Carolina*. Charleston, S.C.: College of Charleston, Center for Metropolitan Affairs and Public Policy, 5-15, 1979.

Kiev, Ari. *Curanderismo: Mexican-American Folk Psychiatry*. New York: The Free Press. 1968.

Kleinman, Arthur. "Medicine's Symbolic Reality: On a Central Problem in the Philosophy of Medicine." *Inquiry*, 16:206-13, 1973.

Kleinman, Arthur. "Concepts and a Model for the Comparison of Medical Systems as Cultural Systems." *Social Science in Medicine*, 12:85-94, 1978.

Kloss, Jethro. *Back to Eden*. Santa Barbara, Cal.: Woodbridge Press Publishing Company, 1972.

Krochmal, Arnold, and Connie Krochmal. *A Guide to Medicinal Plants of the United States*. New York: Quadrangle/The New York Times Book Company, 1975.

Krochmal, Arnold, Russel Walters, and Richard Doughty. *A Guide to Medicinal Plants of Appalachia*. Agriculture Handbook No. 400. Washington, D.C.: Forest Service, U.S. Department of Agriculture, 1969.

Landy, David, "Medical Systems in Transcultural Perspective," in D. Landy, ed., *Culture, Disease and Healing*. New York: Macmillan, 1977.

Leach, Maria, ed. *Funk and Wagnalls Standard Dictionary of Folklore, Mythology, and Legend*. New York: Funk and Wagnalls, 1972.

Lee, John, and Arvilla Payne-Price. "An African-American Folk Healer," in Brett Williams, ed., *The Politics of Culture*. Washington, D.C.: The Smithsonian Institution Press, 155-167, 1991.

List, Paul, and Ludwig Horhammer, eds. *Hagers Handbuch Der Pharmazeutischen Praxis*. Vols. 1-7. Berlin: Springer-Verlag, 1969-79.

Lust, John. *The Herb Book*. New York: Bantam Books/Benedict Lust Publishing, 1974.

Lynas, Lothian. *Medicinal and Food Plants of the North American Indians: A Bibliography*. New York: Library of the New York Botanical Garden, 1972.

Manjo, Guido. *The Healing Hand: Man and Wound in the Ancient World*. Cambridge, Mass.: Harvard University Press, 1975.

Marlowe, Gertrude. "Maggie Lena Walker: African American Women, Business and Community Development," paper presented at The Berkshire Conference on the History of Women, Wellesley, Mass., June 21, 1987.

Mathews, Holly. "Introduction: A Regional Approach and Multidisciplinary Perspective," in Holly Mathews et al., eds., *Traditional Medicine in the South Today*. Durham, N.C: Duke University Press, 1-13, 1992.

Mathews, Holly, James Kirkland, Chip Sullevan, and Karen Baldwin. *Herbal* and *Magical Medicine: Traditional Healing Today.* Durham, N.C.: Duke University Press, 1992.

McQuire, Meredith, with the assistance of Debra Kantor. *Ritual Healing in Suburban America.* New Bruswick, N.J.: Rutgers University Press, 1988.

Meyer, Joseph. *The Herbalist.* Revised and enlarged by Clarence Meyer. Glenwood, Ill.: Meyer Books, 1987.

Miller, Amy. *Shaker Herbs: A History and a Compendium.* New York: Clarkson N. Potter, 1976.

Mitchell, Faith. *Hoodoo Medicine: Sea Islands Herbal Remedies.* Berkeley, Calif: Reed, Cannon and Johnson, 1978.

Mitchell, W. E. "Changing Others: An Anthropological Study of Therapeutic Systems." *Man,* 8: 1977.

Monardes, Nicolas. *Joyfull Newes Out of the Newe Founde Worlde.* London: Da Capo Press, Theatrum Orbis Terravum Ltd., 1577.

Mooney, James. "Cherokee Theory and Practice in Medicine." *Journal of American Folklore,* 3:44-50, 1890.

Mooney, James. *Sacred Formulas of the Cherokees,* 7th Annual Report of the Bureau of American Ethnography, Washington, D.C.: Bureau of American Ethnography, 302-97, 1891.

Mooney, James. *Myths of the Cherokee,* 19th Annual Report of the Bureau of American Ethnography, Washington, D.C.: Bureau of American Ethnography, 3-576, 1900.

Mooney, James. *The Swimmer Manuscript: Cherokee Sacred Formulas and Medicinal Prescriptions.* Revised, completed and edited by F. Olbrechts. Washington, D.C.: U.S. Government Printing Office, 1932.

Morton, Julia. *Folk Remedies of the Low Country.* Miami, Fla.: E. A. Seeman Publishing, 1974.

Morton, Julia. *Major Medicinal Plants: Botany, Culture and Uses.* Springfield, Ill.: Charles C. Thomas, 1977.

Moton, Robert. "Sickness in Slavery Days." *Southern Workman,* 28:74-75, 1899.

Needham, Joseph. *Science and Civilization in China.* 7 Vols. Cambridge: Cambridge University Press, 1954-76.

O'Leary, DeLacy. *How Greek Science Passed to the Arabs.* London: Routledge and K. Paul, 1948.

Otto, John. *Cannon's Point Plantation, 1794-1860: Living Conditions and Status Patterns in the Old South.* New York: Academic Press, 1984.

Payne-Price, Arvilla. "African-American Folk Medicine in the Southeast Lowlands of the United States," in Brett Williams, ed., *The Politics of Culture.* Washington, D.C.: The Smithsonian Institution Press, 133-153, 1991.

Philips, H. Jane. "Lebanese Folk Cures." 2 Vols. Ph.D. Dissertation, Anthropology Department, Columbia University, 1958.

Porcher, Francis. *Resources of the Southern Fields and Forests, Medical, Economical and Agricultural.* Charleston, S.C.: Steam-Pow Press of Evans and Cogswell, 1863.

Postell, William. *The Health of Slaves on Southern Plantations.* Baton Rouge: Louisana State University Press. 1951.

Press, Irwin. "Problems in the Definition and Classification of Medical Systems." *Social Science in Medicine,* 14b:45-57, 1980.

Press, Irwin. "Urban Folk Medicine: A Functional Overview." *American Anthropologist,* 80(1):71-84, 1978.

Primack, Aaron. "The Gospel According to the Voice of Experience," in Lucy Cohen and Tim Ready, eds., *Field Training in Applied Anthropology.* Vol. III. Washington, D.C.: Department of Anthropology, Catholic University of America Press, 55-75, 1984.

Puckett, Newbell. *Folk Beliefs of the Southern Negro.* New York: Negro Universities Press Company, 1968.

Raboteau, Albert. "The Afro-American Traditions," in R. Numbers and D. Amundsen, eds., *Caring and Curing: Health and Medicine in the Western Religous Traditions.* New York: Macmillan, 539-62, 1986.

Readers Digest Association. *Magic and Medicine of Plants.* Pleasantville, N.Y.: Readers Digest Association, 1986.

Rivers, William H. R. *Medicine, Magic and Religion.* New York: Harcourt and Brace, 1924.

Rosengarten, Theodore. *Tombee: Portrait of a Cotton Planter with the Journal of Thomas B. Chaplin (1822-1890).* New York: William Morrow, 1986.

Saunders, L., and G. H. Hewes. "Folk Medicine and Medical Practice," *Journal of Medical Education,* 28(9):43-46, 1953.

Savitt, Todd. *Medicine and Slavery: The Diseases and Health Care of Blacks in Antebellum Virginia.* Chicago: University of Illinois Press, 1978.

Sigerist, Henry. "A History of Medicine." *Primitive and Archaic Medicine.* Vol. 1. New York: Oxford University Press, 1961.

Snow, Loudell. "Folk Medical Beliefs and Their Implications for Care of Patients." *Annals of Internal Medicine,* 81(1):82-96, 1974.

Snow, Loudell. "Popular Medicine in a Black Neigborhood," in E. Spicer, ed., *Ethnic Medicine in the Southwest.* Tuscon: University of Arizona Press, 19-95, 1977.

Snow, Loudell. "Folk Medical Beliefs and Their Implications for the Care of Patients: A Review Based on Studies among Black Americans," in G. Henderson and M. Primeaux, eds., *Transcultural Health Care.* London: Addison-Wesley, 82-96, 1981.

Spector, Rachel. *Cultural Diversity in Health and Illness.* New York: Appleton-Century-Croft, 1979.

Spicer, Edward. *Ethnic Medicine in the Southwest.* Tucson: University of Arizona Press, 1977.

References

Stewart, Horace. "Kindling of Hope in the Disadvantaged: A Study of the Afro-American Healer." *Mental Hygiene,* 55:96-100, 1971.

Sturtevant, William C. "Bibliography of American Indian Medicine and Health." Bureau of American Ethnography March (mimeo), 1962.

Sturtevant, William C. *The Wealth of India: A Dictionary of Indian Raw Materials and Industrial Products.* Vols. 1-10. New Delhi: Publications and Information Directorate, CSIR, 1948.

Swados, F. "Negro Health on the Ante-Bellum Plantations." *Bulletin of the History of Medicine,* 10:460-72, 1941.

Vogel, Virgil. *American Indian Medicine.* Norman: University of Oklahoma Press, 1970.

Watson, Wilbur. *Informal Social Networks in Support of Older Blacks in the Black Belt of the United States.* Washington, D.C.: National Center on Black Aged, 1980.

Watson, Wilbur. *Black Folk Medicine: The Therapeutic Significance of Faith and Trust.* New Brunswick, N.J.: Transaction Books, 1984.

Watt, John, and Maria Breyer-Brandwijk. *The Medicinal and Poisonous Plants of Southern and Eastern Africa.* London: E. and S. Livingstone, Ltd., 1962.

Weiss, Gaea, and Shandor Weiss. *Growing and Using the Healing Herbs.* Emmaus, Penn: Rodale Press, 1985.

White, Newman (ed). *The Frank C. Brown Collection of North Carolina Folklore.* Vols. 6 and 7. Durham, N. C.: Duke University Press, 1961-64.

Wilms, Donald, and W. Powell. *Eastern North Carolina: An Atlas of Demographic and Economic Trends.* Greenville, N.C.: Regional Development Institute of East Carolina University, 1983.

Zimmer, Heinnich. *Hindu Medicine.* Baltimore: Johns Hopkins University Press, 1948.

Index

abortifacient 110
Acorus calamus 36, 37
active ingredients 1, 15, 28, 35
African ix, x, xii, 1-5, 7-12, 14, 17, 19, 21, 23, 25, 27, 32
African American folk medicine xii, 4, 5, 7, 21
ailments 2, 12, 23
Alder Tag 40
allergies 80
Allium sativum 38, 39
Alnus serrulata 40, 41
Aloe 27, 31, 42, 43
Aloe Vera 27, 42, 43
alternative medicine 3, 14
American Indian 7, 8, 17
aphrodisiac 62
Apocynum cannabinum 44, 45
appetite 60, 62, 92, 108, 122
Arctium minus 29, 46, 47
Artemisia absinthium 48, 49
arthritis 23, 25, 29, 32, 44, 62, 80, 92, 104, 112, 122, 150
Asarum virginicum 50, 51
Asclepias spp. 52, 53
asthma 32, 74, 78, 86, 154
astrological sign 25

bad blood 22

Balm 84, 85, 90, 102, 103
Baptisia tinctoria 54, 55
bark 1, 28, 29, 40, 88, 114, 126, 128, 130, 152
Bear's foot 123
bedwetting 156
Bee Balm 102, 103
bile 8, 24
binary qualities 21
biomedicine 3, 4, 14, 26
bitter 11, 19, 25, 29, 48, 62, 72, 86
Black Cherry 126
Black Cohosh 29, 31, 32, 62, 63
Black Nightshade 144
Black Snakeroot 136, 137
bladder 92
blood 7, 13, 21-24, 30, 38, 44, 48, 62, 64, 80, 92, 108, 130, 138, 148
blood cells 24
blood purifier 30, 44, 62
blood purity 21, 22
bloodletting 8, 9
boils 92, 159
Boneset 72, 73
botanical repertoire 27
bowel problems 138
bronchitis 19, 62

bruises 54, 116
Burdock 29, 46, 47
burns 13, 42

cancer 40, 100, 112, 120, 150
canker sores 46
carminative 102
Cassia marilandica 56, 57
catching the spirit 10
Catnip 18, 28, 29, 104, 105
caul 18
chemical potency 29
Chenopodium 58, 59
chicken pox 86, 104, 134
Chimaphila maculata 60, 61
Chinaberry 88, 89
Cimicifuga racemosa 29, 31, 32, 62, 63
circulation 21-24, 48, 64
Citrullus lanatus 64, 65
clairvoyance 25
classification 5, 27, 28, 32, 35
colds 19, 22, 23, 25, 30, 38, 46, 66, 72, 78, 86, 104, 106, 114, 126, 134, 138, 154
colic 36, 100, 104, 159
conjure doctors 9, 10
conjuring 9, 10
constipation 80, 112, 140, 148
consumption 38, 108
Corn silk 156, 157
cough 24, 38, 114, 159
Cynoglossum virginianum 66, 67
cysts 30, 112

Dandelion 29, 148, 149
dandruff 50, 92, 122
Datura stramonium 28, 70, 71
Daucus carota 68, 69
diabetes 22, 29, 54, 62, 76, 92, 108, 120, 122, 148
diagnostic system 5, 2, 4, 21
diaper rash 104

divine intervention 13
Dog Nettle 142, 143
dreams 13, 25, 26

ear infection 31
Eastern White Pine 114
emphysema 38
etiologies 7
Eupatorium perfoliatum 72, 73
Euphorbia hirta 74, 75
European colonial 7
European Pennyroyal 100
evil spirits 10

faith healers 13
falling out 22
fever 8, 18, 22, 62, 104, 122, 159
fix 13, 15, 19, 25, 30
Flagroot 36
flashes 22, 25
flu 72, 114
fluid 31, 72
Fly Weed 58, 59
folk practitioners 2
folk psychiatrist 12
folk wisdom 1, 4, 32
fungal 112

gall 24
Gall-of-the-Earth 44, 45
Garlic 38, 39
gas 36, 68, 102, 104
Gaylussacia spp. 76, 77
genera 9, 27, 33
Ginseng 30, 108, 109
Gnaphalium obtusifolium 78, 79
God 10, 13, 19, 25
Golden Seal 30, 80, 81
good blood 22
gout 46, 66, 80, 92
granny midwife 11
Grip Grass 28, 140, 141

Index

harmful 28, 35
Hazel Alder 40
headaches 78, 134
Heart Leaf 50, 51
heart murmur 92
heart trouble 60, 62
heartburn 36
hemorrhoids 128, 130, 154
herbal practitioner 7
herbal remedies 9, 10, 18, 19, 28
herbalist 1, 5, 11, 12, 17
high blood pressure 22, 38
hives 104
hoarseness 126
hoodoo 10
hooting owl 25, 26
Horehound 86, 87
Horse Nettle 142
Horsemint 96, 97
Housemint 98, 99
howling dog 25, 26
Huckleberry 76, 77
humors of the body 7, 21
Hydrastis canadensis 80, 81

impetigo 112
impurities in blood 22, 24, 30, 31
indigestion 25, 36, 48, 126
insect bites 52, 54, 144
insomnia 90, 104

Jimsonweed 28, 70, 71

kidney problems 92, 108, 122, 128, 138, 148

Lactuca spp. 82, 83
laxative 28, 56
laying-on-of-hands 13
Lemon Mint 90, 91
Leonurus cardiaca 84, 85
liver 22, 24, 38, 108, 128, 148, 150

location 4, 21, 22, 28
loss of appetite 62, 92, 122
low blood pressure 92

Maggie Walker 11
magic 7, 9, 10, 13, 17, 26
magic vendor 13
magical charms 10
magical medicine 10
malaria 8, 15, 130
Male Fern 124, 125
Marrubium vulgare 86, 87
materia medica 1, 2, 5, 9, 12, 27, 29, 32
Mayapple 118, 119
measles 19, 114
medical botanicals 8, 27
Melia azedarach 88, 89
Melissa officinalis 90, 91
Menispermum canadense 29, 31, 32, 92
menstrual cramps 36, 62, 66, 68, 102, 104, 134, 146
Mentha pulegium 100, 101
Mentha spp. 94-99
midwives 1, 11-13, 15, 18
Milkweed 52, 53, 74, 75, 82, 83
Mint 94, 95
Mistletoe 110, 111
Monarda didyma 102, 103
moonseed 92
mother wit 1, 4, 32
Motherwort 84, 85
mouth sores 132
mucus 78
Mullein 154, 155
mumps 156, 160

natural illness 10
nausea 102
neighborhood prophets 13
Nepeta cataria 18, 28, 29, 104, 105

nerves 24, 108
nervousness 102
Nightshade 18, 28, 31, 144, 145

occult illness 10
odor 29
Oenothera biennis 106, 107
old-home remedies 2, 18

Panax quinquefolius 108, 109
Pennyroyal 9, 33, 100, 101
pharmacopoeia ix, x, 2, 8, 11, 27, 29
phlegm 8, 21, 24
Phoradendron serotinum 110, 111
Phytolacca americana 28-30, 112, 113
Pigweed 120, 121
Pinkweed 120
Pinus strobus 29, 30, 114, 115
plant 19, 28, 29, 86, 112
Plantago major 27, 28, 116, 117
Plantain 27, 28, 116, 117
plantations 8, 9, 11
pluralistic 4
pneumonia 8, 72, 114, 159
Podophyllum peltatum 118, 119
Poison Ivy 18, 52, 144
Poison Oak 52
poisonous x, 28, 29, 35
Poke Root 28-30, 112, 113
Pokeweed 112
Polygonum pennsylvanica 120, 121
Polymnia uvedalia 29, 32, 122, 123
Polystichum acrostichoides 124, 125
possession 10, 19
powerful 28, 29, 35, 48, 58, 70, 100, 110, 112, 144
practitioners 1, 2, 4, 9, 11-13
prayers 13
Primrose (Evening) 106, 107

prostate gland 62, 92, 108, 122, 159
Prunus serotina 126, 127
purging 8

quantitative efficacy 28
quantity of blood 21, 22, 40
Queen Anne's lace 69
Quercus alba 29, 128, 129
Quercus rubra 29, 130, 131

Rabbit Tobacco 28, 78, 79
rash 30, 31, 104
Rat's Vein 61
Red Bergamot 102, 103
Red Clover 150, 151
Red Oak bark 29, 130
Red Sumac 132, 133
religion 7, 10, 14
religious rituals 10
rheumatism 46, 62
Rhus glabra 132, 133
root doctors 1, 10, 13, 15, 18
rooted by magic 25

Sage 134, 135
Salvia officinalis 134, 135
Sanicula marilandica 136, 137
Sarsaparilla 29, 31, 32, 92
Sassafras 138, 139
Sassafras albidium 138, 139
Sea Islands 12
seasonal change 23
seasonal forces 29
seed ticks 100
Senna 56, 57
shouting churches 10
sinus 80
Sisyrinchium spp. 140, 141
slavery 8, 10, 11
slaves 8-12, 15, 27
sleep 29
Slippery Elm 152, 153

Index

Smooth Sumac 132
Solanum carolinense 142, 143
Solanum nigrum 18, 144, 145
sorcery 10
sore throat 38, 154
sores 22, 44, 46, 52, 70, 74, 82, 116, 132, 136, 138, 154
Spearmint 98, 99
spirit possession 10
spiritual illness 10, 13
Spotted Pipsissewa 60
spring tonic 112, 138
stomach troubles 42, 94, 96, 98
styes 92
supernatural healing 2
Sweet Flag 36
swelling 46, 54, 62, 66, 92, 100, 116, 122, 138, 154, 160
symbolism 26
symptoms 21, 22, 26

talk-off-warts 13
talk-out-bleeding 13, 18
talk-out-fire 13, 18
Tanacetum vulgare 146, 147
Tansy 146, 147
Taraxacum officinale 29, 148, 149
taste 28, 29, 35
temperature 21, 23, 24
therapists 11
therapy 2, 4, 7, 8, 28, 32
thick/thin blood 21, 23, 24
thrush 104
thyroid 112
tired blood 24
toxic 28
Trifolium pratense 150, 151
tumors 106

ulcers 36, 66, 112
Ulmus rubra 152, 153
unnatural illness 10
upset stomach 36

urinary tract 44, 64, 84, 92, 148
urinary tract infection 64, 84

varicose veins 29, 46, 128, 130
veil 18
Verbascum thapsus 154, 155
viscosity 21, 23
visions 22
voodoo 7, 10, 14

warts 13, 74, 82, 154
wasp stings 52, 144, 159
Watermelon seeds 64
weak eyes 92
whistling bird 25
White Oak bark 29, 128
White Pine Top 114, 115
Wild Cherry 126, 127
Wild Comfrey 29, 66, 67
Wild Indigo 54, 55
Wild Lettuce 82, 83
Wild Senna 56
witchcraft 10
worldview 10
worms 36, 88, 124, 128
Wormwood 48, 49
wounds 66, 128, 132, 154

Zea mays 156, 157

About the Author

ARVILLA PAYNE-JACKSON is Associate Professor, Department of Sociology and Anthropology, Howard University. An expert on African American herbal medicine, she collaborates in this book with John Lee, a well-known herbalist who practices in North Carolina and lectures widely.